Therapeutic Uses of *Music* with Older Adults

Alicia Ann Clair
Jenny Memmott

Second Edition

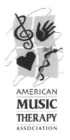

AMERICAN
MUSIC
THERAPY
ASSOCIATION

	Second Edition
ISBN:	978-1-884914-03-4
Authors:	Alicia Ann Clair, PhD, MT-BC
	Jenny Memmott
Copyright Information:	©American Music Therapy Association, Inc. 2008
	8455 Colesville Road, Suite 1000
	Silver Spring, MD 20910 USA
	www.musictherapy.org
	info@musictherapy.org

Cover design and Layout:	Tawna Grasty, Grass T Design
Technical Assistance:	Wordsetters
	Kalamazoo, Michigan

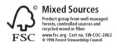

Printed in the United States of America

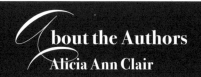

About the Authors
Alicia Ann Clair

Alicia Ann Clair, PhD, MT-BC, is a professor, division director of music education and music therapy, and a faculty affiliate of the gerontology center at the University of Kansas where she teaches music therapy courses for both undergraduate and graduate students.

Dr. Clair is a music therapy practitioner and clinical researcher who has specialized in music therapy practice with persons who have diagnoses of Alzheimer's Disease or related dementias and their professional and family caregivers since 1988, and with persons who are well, older adults, and older adults with disabilities since 1975. She participates as a Research Associate at the Eastern Kansas Veterans Administration Health Care System, Topeka Campus where she regularly conducts clinical sessions and practice research.

Dr. Clair is a member of a national Veterans Administration workgroup to develop treatment approaches in transitional rehabilitation for Operation Iraqi Freedom (OIF) and Operation Enduring Freedom (OEF) military personnel who have experienced combat injuries.

She is a past President of the American Music Therapy Association and was awarded the National Service Award, the National Professional Practices Award, the National Research Award, and an honorary life membership award by that organization.

She is the author of many scholarly publications and has presented clinical protocols and clinical research outcomes throughout the world.

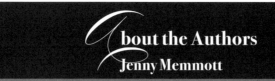

About the Authors
Jenny Memmott

Jenny Memmott is a graduate student in music therapy at the University of Kansas. During her music therapy clinical training, Ms. Memmott worked with individuals with developmental disabilities, teenagers with emotional and behavioral disorders, older adults, and hospice patients and their families. She co-authored a major research study, "Examination of Relationships between Participation in School Music Programs of Differing Quality and Standardized Test Results," which was published in the Winter 2006 edition of the *Journal of Music Education*. She received her B.A. in English from the University of Kansas.

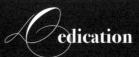

Dedication

*This book is dedicated to all those who work to improve the
life quality of older adults and their families.*

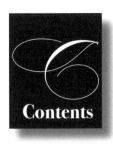

Contents

Preface

This book has been updated with the latest information available concerning the use of music with older adults. It was written for all those who want to use music to improve life quality in older adults whether they are family, professionals, friends or older persons themselves. The book contains practical applications of music that can be readily used, even by persons who have minimal or no music education, training, or experience. While the book gives some guidance for beginning music therapy practitioners in the field of gerontology, it is truly intended for all those who understand the role of music as a wonderful and powerful influence in life.

This book does not provide a detailed set of protocols that constitute step-by-step sequences of techniques that lead to predictable outcomes. Instead it gives a theoretical basis for using music and gently guides the reader to draw on available resources to contribute to life quality in older adults through music.

The information presented through this book is not intended to take the place of a professionally trained, board certified music therapist. There is no substitute for a qualified music therapy practitioner when assessment, treatment design, implementation, and evaluation are required to restore physical, cognitive, or psychosocial functioning.

It is sincerely hoped that the information presented within can make music more accessible to all those who are interested, willing, and committed to using it to bring better life quality to persons in their later years. Best wishes and good luck!

Chapter 1

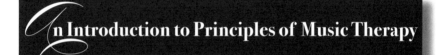

n Introduction to Principles of Music Therapy

An Introduction to Principles of Music Therapy

Music therapy is a relatively new field among contemporary therapeutic disciplines. Although music has been used in medicine since the beginning of recorded history, and most likely even earlier (Davis & Gfeller, 1999), current applications are innovative. The principles upon which music therapy is based, however, are rooted in a long history of successful applications. The first of these applications described in the English language appeared as a monograph written by a London apothecary named Richard Browne, probably in the early 1600s, and published posthumously in 1729 (Gibbons & Heller, 1985). Browne articulated several principles that are among those upon which current music therapy practices are based. These principles include the following:

1. The influence of stimulative and sedative music on human responses, including psychological responses

2. The power of music to evoke associations and memories

3. The power of music to influence moods

4. The associations between emotions and psychosomatic disorders

5. The use of music in preventive health care

6. The possibility of some music, or some uses of music, having deleterious effects

7. The use of participation in music for positive effects on the whole person

8. The therapeutic success with music, which depends not upon the consumer's musical training but upon appropriate adjustment to the consumer's ability and function levels.

Furthermore, a respected 18th-century British physician by the name of Richard Brocklesby wrote a treatise entitled *Reflections on the Power of Music*, in which Brocklesby theorized that the application of music could cure certain illnesses and disorders (Brocklesby, 1749). The first published article concerning the therapeutic uses of music in the United States appeared in 1789, the same year George Washington was elected President (Heller, 1987). It was followed by a second publication in 1796 and by additional works in the 1800s that claimed beneficial effects of music on various health problems, including mania, depression, and pain, and in the education of students at the Perkins School for the Blind in Boston (Heller, 1987).

These early works began to capture attention concerning the therapeutic uses of music, but writings about the treatment of physical ailments and mental disorders using music were slow to emerge. The body of literature began to develop in the United States during the 19th century. The articles that appeared in American medical journals, psychiatric periodicals, and medical dissertations described music as an alternative, holistic approach to medical treatment (Davis, 1987). Although these writings were based largely on isolated anecdotal reports and little empirical research, they marked the beginnings of contemporary music therapeutic practice.

In the early years of the 20th century, music therapy evolved as a viable therapeutic modality, largely through the efforts of three women: Eva Augusta Vescelius, Isa Maud Ilsen, and Harriet Ayer Seymour (Davis, 1993). The work of these women was so noteworthy that they were recognized by the American Red Cross and the U.S. Army. However, the skepticism of the general public and a lack of formal structure caused the failure of the music therapy organizations they founded (Davis & Gfeller, 1999). Nevertheless, these women were the first Americans to practice clinical music therapy for extended periods of time, and upon their practical experience they based empirical research concerning the therapeutic effects of music. They used their practical experience and research knowledge to develop philosophies of treatment and to train musicians in the proper applications of music for children and adults in hospitals, asylums, prisons, and schools (Davis, 1993).

The work of these early music therapy pioneers was handed down to the musicians they trained. By the outbreak of World War II, music was integrated into rehabilitation for soldiers injured in battle. The military encouraged the use of music, particularly to lift morale (Boxberger, 1963), and musicians began to implement diversionary and other music activities for the soldiers. With the success of the military programs, music applications spread to civilian hospitals, and professional music associations provided the instruments, supplies, and leadership that supported these hospital programs. The demand for therapeutic music services grew, as did the demand for training. Michigan State University implemented the first degree program in 1944, which was followed by four others in the next two years, including the University of Kansas, Lawrence; Chicago Musical College; College of the Pacific, Stockton, California; and Alverno College, Milwaukee (Boxberger, 1963). The field was quickly emerging and there was a great need to provide communication, organization, and leadership to the many people engaged in the uses of music in hospitals. To meet this need, the National Association for Music Therapy (NAMT) was established in 1950. The American Association for Music Therapy (AAMT) was founded in 1971. In 1998, the National Association for Music Therapy united with the American Association for Music Therapy to become the American Music Therapy Association, or AMTA.

Through the years, the practice of music therapy has evolved as the needs for interventions have changed. The AMTA continues to provide support for practitioners in the field through its publication of two nationally refereed professional journals, an annual conference, legislative activities at both federal and state levels, networking among members and among other professional associations, public and professional education, any many other professional activities.

DEFINITION OF MUSIC THERAPY

The AMTA has defined music therapy as follows:

Music Therapy is the clinical and evidence-based use of music interventions to accomplish individualized goals within a therapeutic relationship by a credentialed professional who has completed an approved music therapy program. (AMTA, 2006b, p. 19)

The AMTA (2007) has further defined music therapy as an effective treatment option for older persons:

Music therapy treatment is efficacious and valid for older persons who have functional deficits in physical, psychological, cognitive and social functioning. Research results and clinical experiences attest to the viability of music therapy even in those who are resistive to other treatment approaches. Music is a form of sensory stimulation, which provokes responses due to the familiarity, predictability, and feelings of security associated with it.

A definition of music therapy is difficult to articulate because it draws upon many disciplines associated with both music and therapy (Bruscia, 1998). In addition, music therapy programming is designed to meet the specific needs of individuals and to help them achieve specific goals. Music therapy also has the component of a trained music therapist who provides the expertise needed for proper program design, implementation, and evaluation. Ultimately music therapy includes the application of music by a credentialed music therapy professional that is time-limited and guided by goals and objectives derived from ongoing assessment and evaluation of a person's functional levels.

The goals of music therapy programs are focused on remediation of individual needs and the development of nonmusical skills and abilities that facilitate the best possible function in the least restrictive community. These programs incorporate music and the medium for therapeutic intervention, but the outcomes are clearly nonmusical. Musical products such as performances, recordings, songs written, or music composed during the course of the program are not the purpose of the intervention, but are merely the vehicles through which other outcomes are achieved (e.g., improved cognitive function through increased sustained, alternating and divided attention; increased verbal engagement in social interactions; increased range of motion and physical strength or flexibility obtained by increased adherence to exercise regimens; decreased symptoms of depression; better sleep hygiene; improved stress and pain management).

Although music therapists do not implement programs with the purpose of developing musical products, any participation in music must include the best musical achievement possible. The quality of all musical experiences in the course of the intervention is important because it is associated directly with accomplishment and satisfaction. When the musical experiences are unsuccessful, of poor quality, or judged to be unsatisfying by the participants, little probability exists that participants will continue to engage, and, if participation does not continue, there is little chance of meeting the needs of the individual participants. Satisfaction with the musical experience is the motivating force for continued commitment to the therapeutic process. Music therapists, therefore, design music therapy applications that provide experiences that are desirable, motivating, and appropriate for program participants. These applications are viable and efficacious over a broad range of skills and abilities in older people. A background in music is not a prerequisite for successful experiences (*Forever Young: Music and Aging*, 1991). The skills required of music therapists in order to develop and implement successful music experiences, which are integral to the therapeutic process, are acquired in professional education and training.

QUALIFICATIONS OF A MUSIC THERAPIST

Individuals who have completed necessary coursework from a professionally approved college or university music therapy program and who have completed a music therapy internship at an approved site are eligible to take a national certification board examination to earn the credential of Music Therapist–Board Certified (MT-BC). This examination, which is administered and maintained by the Certification Board for Music Therapists (CBMT), assesses whether the therapist demonstrates entry-level skills for the profession (AMTA, 2006a, p. xi). These certified professionals have multidisciplinary backgrounds that include music, behavioral and social sciences, liberal arts and sciences, and music therapy theory and clinical practice.

DESIGN AND IMPLEMENTATION OF A
MUSIC THERAPY PROGRAM

When a qualified music therapist designs an individual therapy program, he or she must consider both music as therapy and music in therapy (Bruscia, 1998). *Music as therapy* is the full integration of music into an intervention. In this case, music is so essential to the intervention that lesser results, or no results at all, occur when music is excluded. With older adults, this can mean an inability to function, or at least an inability to function well, without music as part of the intervention. This is exemplified by the client who has an uneven ambulatory gait. Using music with enhanced beats, the client can learn to walk with a more even stride (Clair & O'Konski, 2006; Hamburg

& Clair, 2003; Thaut, McIntosh, Prassas, & Rice, 1992, 1993). People with Alzheimer's disease or dementia who can no longer carry on conversations can interact with one another and with others nonverbally by playing rhythms using percussion instruments (Cevasco & Grant, 2006; Clair, 1991a, 1991b, 2002b, 2002c; Clair & Bernstein, 1990a, 1990b; Clair, Bernstein, & Johnson, 1995; Groene, 2001), or they may dance ballroom style with a partner (Clair, 2002a; Clair & Ebberts, 1997; Clair, Tebb, & Bernstein, 1993). In all these examples, music is essential to the therapeutic processes. Without music, the responses are no longer possible, or, at best, they are greatly diminished.

With *music in therapy*, it is the inherent qualities of the music that facilitate achieving therapeutic outcomes. The music enhances therapeutic approaches, but it may not be the only medium that can yield desirable results. Other interventions may lead to the same treatment outcomes, but music may be the medium of choice. In this context, music may promote relaxation for anxious or agitated people by providing a structured, predictable environment. Music may be used to focus and train sustained attention. Music may also alter moods, evoke a desirable emotion, stimulate a memory for reminiscence, stimulate verbal expressions of feelings that range from anger and frustration to joy and satisfaction, or provide the aesthetic enjoyment that is so essential to quality of life.

Whether music is used as therapy or in therapy, the music therapist's role is to design and implement individualized music therapy program plans based on initial and ongoing assessments of clients' functions. Music therapists use assessments to target treatment needs and they seek input from the client, the client's family, or both to determine treatment plan priorities. Once implemented, the outcomes of the individualized plan are determined through the ongoing assessments of progress toward treatment objectives. Assessment information is shared with the client, the client's family, and other professionals associated with the client's treatment. The assessment outcomes are used as evidence that the planned program is effective or requires change. The program is subsequently maintained or altered accordingly. The assessment and evaluation of an individual's program participation is ongoing and is monitored carefully to assure appropriate evidence-based outcomes.

THERAPEUTIC OUTCOMES OF MUSIC

The definition of what is and is not therapeutic must be made in the context of an individual's specific needs. What is therapeutic is defined by what treats or cures diseases or disorders, rehabilitates, maintains or restores health, or benefits one's mental state. Within this framework, music is therapeutic in older individuals when it provides relief from physical, social, or emotional discomfort, and when it contributes to their ability to function.

Music is therefore therapeutic when it contributes to improvements in physical, cognitive, social, and/or emotional functions. In turn, therapeutic outcomes are judged by their contributions to an individual's integration into community, whatever it may be, and the life quality that results.

It is important to note that therapeutic outcomes do not depend on universally effective prescriptive approaches, but are individually designed in content and scope by a professionally trained music therapist. Clients are not forced into a therapeutic mold; rather, the therapeutic approach is shaped and adapted specifically for each client. The approach must actualize the desires of the individual and the individual's family or guardian, and it must comply with standards of professional practice and ethics (Clair, 1994).

Evidence-based Music Therapy Practice

Evidence-based practice has become the guide to treatment in music therapy. Evidence-based practice is an outgrowth of evidence-based medicine in which reliable and practical research is used to inform health care decisions. The focus on research evidence in medical decisions was a reaction to criticisms of traditional clinical authority as the guide to practice. Furthermore, the escalating costs of medical care forced care providers to demonstrate which services are necessary for health and which services are of little or no health benefit (Shapiro, Laskerk, Bindman, & Lee,1993). The result was an explosion of scientific studies, the development of clinical skills to assess and use the information taken from the research, and the application of this information to achieve the best possible outcomes (Daly, 2005).

Initially, the study of health outcomes, which began about 30 years ago, incorporated physiological measures as indicators for intervention use and for determining intervention success, but researchers found that physiological measures alone missed the factors that mattered most to people—their ability to function and their quality of life (United States National Library of Medicine, 2004). Furthermore, measures of factors related to persons' lives, including social contexts where patients make decisions regarding compliance with treatment regimens, have become important (Daly, 2005). The complex issues associated with evidence-based medicine leads to multidisciplinary collaboration, including music therapy, where problems are identified, research methods are selected, and the best outcomes are achieved (Daly, 2005). The need for evidence-based outcomes in music therapy has become essential in the effort to demonstrate accountability for intervention results.

GUIDING PRINCIPLES FOR USING MUSIC THERAPEUTICALLY

Pervasiveness of Music

One of the factors that makes music an attractive medium for therapeutic interventions is its pervasiveness. Most people experience music frequently, many on a daily basis. Some people listen to music virtually all day. Music is almost always used in the celebrations and rituals associated with important life events, such as birthdays, anniversaries, weddings, and funerals; in the work environment; in entertainment; and in structuring leisure time. Such pervasive uses for music in the world have led anthropologist Alan Merriam (1964) to conclude that no other known cultural activity reaches into, shapes, and controls so much of human behavior as does music.

The frequent uses of music have led many people to refer to it as a universal phenomenon. In fact, there is no known culture that does not have music as an art form (Nettl, 1956). Although some musical elements, such as rhythm, tempo, and timbre, are found universally, the types of music preferred, understood, and used are not the same for all people in all cultures (Gfeller, 2002b). The music from one culture may not be understood or even tolerated by another culture. Differences exist even in the same culture when the preferences of the old and the young are compared. Differences in preference have often been an issue between adolescents and their parents, and the differences can be even more extreme between adolescents and their grandparents. The types of music within a community or even within a family from that community may vary according to age, background, and experience. Therefore, music is universal, but it is not a universal language.

Musical Preference

A person's preference for a particular type or types of music depends on familiarity. Musical preference is, therefore, associated with age, cultural group, and peer group. Because these preferences result from experience and familiarity, they are a function of learning (Radocy & Boyle, 2003). Thus, preferred music is music that is most often used by people and is well integrated into their lives. This music could be that which was popular during their young adult years (Flowers & Murphy, 2001; Gibbons, 1977; Jonas, 1991), that which is used in religious services and patriotic ceremonies, or that which is used in other cultural and community contexts (Lathom, Peterson, & Havlicek, 1982). Music that is not integrated into a person's life may simply have no effect on that individual or may even be offensive, resulting in inattention, agitation, or disengagement.

People may prefer different types of music at different life periods, and as they gain musical experience, they may broaden their musical tastes and preferences. For example, some people may have liked rock and roll music in their young adult years. Although they still listen to it later in life, they may also have expanded their musical tastes to include various types of jazz, some classical music, and rhythm and blues. The same people may also learn to use certain types of music for particular purposes in therapeutic interventions, such as relaxation and stress management. It may be possible, therefore, for someone who prefers listening to rock music to use classical music in a music therapy intervention.

In order for interventions to be efficacious, it is important to determine the preferred music for individual clients. It is the preferred music that is more likely to encourage participation and commitment to the treatment regimen, at least initially. Although many types of music may elicit responses, it is the music with which individuals are familiar that seems to have the greatest potential to evoke emotional reactions and, subsequently, motivate participation (Thaut, 2002).

The type or types of preferred music used in music therapy interventions may be determined by interviewing clients or their family members if clients can no longer express themselves verbally. If interview responses are inconclusive or unavailable, it is possible to determine music preferences by using various types of music and observing reactions to the music. Facial expressions, body postures, vocalizations, and other overt responses to particular pieces of music indicate pleasure, apathy, or even discomfort associated with the music.

Using Music Therapeutically with Older Adults

Music Provides Physical and Emotional Stimulation

Music can be used with older people to evoke wide ranges of physical responses. Depending upon how it is structured, music can be sedative (to promote relaxation and calm) or stimulative (to promote movement or other physical activity).

A review of the literature indicates clearly that the definitions of sedative and stimulative music are individualized and that no consistent agreement exists among listeners (Hodges, 1980). What may be calming and quieting to one person may be disturbing and disquieting to another. Individuals with whom the music is used must determine its sedative or stimulative effects. Generally, sedative music tends to have no accented beats, no percussive characteristics, no syncopation (Gaston, 1968), slow tempos, and smooth melodic contours. If the music is instrumental, the predominant instruments are strings and woodwinds. Stimulative music generally tends to have accented beats, percussive characteristics, syncopation (Gaston, 1968), fast tempos, and smooth or nonsmooth melodic contours. If the music is instrumental, the predominant instruments are most often percussion, brass, and bass.

The sedative or stimulative qualities of music evoke not only calm or activity but other physiological responses as well. Research with subjects over a wide range of ages has shown that music can affect blood pressure, heart rate, respiration, galvanic (excited) skin response, pupil dilation, discomfort, and tolerance to pain (Malone,

1996; Standley, 1986, 1992; Whitehead-Pleaux, Baryza, & Sheridan, 2006). These reactions to music differ from individual to individual, but there is no question that music has a powerful influence over physiological responses. It may be that these physical reactions are the bases for quieting responses to sedative music and for activating responses to stimulative music,

In addition to the physical responses associated with sedative and simulative music, evidence exists that physical responses are tied to emotional reactions. The power of music to influence mood and affect is represented well throughout the literature (Hodges, 1980; Radocy & Boyle, 2003). Clinical observations and research have further shown that physiological responses to music are also integral to emotional responses (Thaut, 2002). Therefore, a particular emotion can be triggered by certain music for a certain individual, and clinical observations show that this individual's emotional, reaction to specific music is relatively consistent. These emotional reactions can be either pleasant or unpleasant, very intense or quite mild.

Once these specific emotional reactions in an individual are known, music can be used to facilitate a transition from a deleterious emotional reaction to a more productive one. Music also may be used to stimulate someone who is otherwise disengaged or unresponsive.

Music Facilitates Social Interaction

All humans have the need to belong, to be a part of a group of individuals who share and who come together for a common purpose (Gaston, 1968; Gfeller, 2002b). This need for connection with others may be the most important component of quality of life (Roskam, 1993). Although humans have this need, they may not possess the ability or capacity to meet it themselves. They may lack social skills, or they may not possess the emotional characteristics that attract other people. They may have physical limitations that are the result of frailty, illness, or financial circumstances that restrict their access to opportunities to interact with other people. They may have cognitive losses associated with dementia or other impairments that restrict or prohibit meaningful interactions. People who perceive themselves to be fully functional may also not know how to relate to people who seem not to be fully functional, and may even react with discomfort when confronted with them. In order to avoid discomfort, functional people avoid confrontation, and, consequently, people with physical or mental limitations are abandoned and become even more isolated.

This abandonment has far-reaching effects. It occurs not only with the individual who has become dysfunctional through disease, injury, or other means, but also with the individual's spouse and family. Whether gradual or sudden, the invitations extended to these caregivers to participate in social events diminish greatly or may cease altogether. This exclusion may occur because these people are so tied to their caregiving responsibilities that their time and availability are severely restricted. As a result, they turn down so many social opportunities that they are eliminated from invitation on the assumption that they will refuse to participate. Eventually they are excluded from all social activity in which they once participated. They find themselves alone, burdened, and bound to the demands of caregiving, with no way to reach out to other people.

As people who are engaged in caregiving are abandoned, so are people for whom status has changed through divorce, serious illness or injury, or the death of a spouse or a close companion. These individuals may find themselves left alone by friends, who may tell them to telephone if they need anything, but who do not continue making contact. It seems these "friends" may use avoidance to relieve their own discomfort associated with loss through death or other means. They find it impossible to continue interacting with people who are in painful circumstances, and they may not relate comfortably to people who have experienced a change in status even after they have adjusted to their new lives. The network of friends and acquaintances therefore disintegrates.

A need for intervention exists for people who want to belong with others but cannot do so, either through their own limitations or the limitations on the people around them. Music therapy is one intervention that can draw people together because they enjoy music and generally enjoy their experiences with it. People feel comfortable with music, especially when it is familiar, and they can feel secure in the predictable structure it provides. Music also provides opportunities for common experiences, which are the basis for relationships. Participating in music provides social interaction by using a medium that is nonthreatening. It is usually not possible to talk about personal issues that may be uncomfortable while performing or listening to music, but sharing music can often lead to sharing other life experiences. For example, people who make music together may travel together to and from rehearsals, and people who listen to music may attend musical events with one another. They may continue to socialize after the musical experience and they may share some things about their personal lives. Whenever such sharing becomes uncomfortable, discussions can shift to music topics and to making plans for future events. Here, sharing the music provides the basis and the reason for social interaction.

Music Provides Communication

As with all art forms, music is communicative (Gaston, 1968; Gfeller, 2002c.) What it conveys is unique. It cannot be done better in any way or through any other medium. This communication may occur verbally, through lyrics in a melodic context, or nonverbally, relying totally upon one or more musical elements. The potential for communication makes using music viable for people who are nonverbal or who have communication deficits in order to facilitate their social interactions. Music may be the only medium through which some of these people can interact and have some sense that they belong. The following example illustrates this point:

> Mrs. Jackson has late-stage dementia. She has not spoken in several years, and can no longer walk because of the progression of the disease. Although Mrs. Jackson generally does not make vocal sounds, she does make a vocal response at specific points each time a certain song is sung to her. History provided by family members indicates that the song is familiar and that she enjoyed singing it early in her life. Mrs. Jackson makes ongoing attempts to sing, even though she can no longer match the pitches or articulate the lyrics.

Mrs. Jackson can still enter into some level of participation with others because the structure of the familiar song makes it possible for her to use residual abilities in order to respond vocally, and do so in a rhythmic and melodic context. The music provides the opportunities to interact meaningfully with others and to be socially integrated. Most of all, music makes it possible for her to escape the isolation of degenerative disease, if only for a short time.

Music Provides Emotional Expression

Because music can be used to communicate nonverbally, it is particularly helpful as an emotional outlet for people who have limited or no verbal communication skills. Music also enhances emotional expression for people who can articulate their feelings. For both verbal and nonverbal people, music may be used to express a wide variety of emotions, from anger and frustration to affection and tenderness. These expressions can take the form of vocalizations, which may or may not require words, or the form of playing an instrument, physical movement, or facial expression.

Musical expression may serve as an iconic representation of an individual's emotions (Gfeller, 2002a). For example, people whose loved ones have been diagnosed with a serious illness for which the prognosis for recovery is poor usually experience terrible anger and feelings of helplessness, at least initially. When involved in music therapy applications that incorporate percussive instruments, these people hit drums with great force and loudness, while their facial expressions reveal knitted brows, tense facial muscles, pursed lips, and tight jaws. The effect they experience may not be verbalized, but their observable behaviors with music indicate expressions of strong emotions. These observations may be used to stimulate discussions about the emotions people feel or as an opportunity to vent their emotions in socially appropriate and nonthreatening ways.

Music Evokes Associations

One aspect that makes music unique is the associations each person makes with particular selections (Gfeller, 2002c). The associations may be with times, places, or people. These associations may evoke emotions, visual images, or other sensory information, including perceptions of flavors, odors, textures, temperatures, comforts, and discomforts, and may be either direct or indirect. In other words, the music may have been heard in only one context or situation and hearing it evokes a specific memory of that situation. The music may also have a certain style that is generally associated with a period of time in one's life, and hearing any music in that style stimulates memories of that time. These memories or associations may evoke happiness, sadness, or even remorse. They are also so individual that they are impossible to predict—a song that evokes smiles and apparent happiness for one person may trigger tears and apparent grief for another. For example, for one person, a big band tune may elicit a smile and reminiscences of delightful times dancing at the local ballroom as a young adult. The same song may cause another person to become tearful, as he or she remembers a young person who went off to war and never came back. As with music preference, some information about a person's reactions to certain music is helpful. It is also important to observe behavioral indications of reactions, whether verbal or nonverbal.

With such strong associations, music is often used as a stimulus for reminiscence and life review in older people, but it can serve the same purpose in people of all ages. The music that was a part of an individual's experience during his or her lifetime can be selected for reminiscence. Clinical observations show that music facilitates discussion of the past, and even when individuals cannot respond verbally because of physical or mental disabilities, they can sometimes sing the songs that were part of their life before the disability. When these singing skills cannot be employed because of the disease or illness, a person can continue to enjoy listening to the songs. Music can still simulate positive experiences, either through evoking fond memories and positive feelings or through providing comfort through predictability and familiarity.

Music Provides Diversion from Inactivity, Discomfort, and Daily Routine

Some older people have great amounts of available time with nothing to fill it. There may be hours in every day in which there is nothing to do, either because of frailty, the lack of other people, financial limitations, or other circumstances. Described by some as the worst possible condition under which to live, unfilled time leaves people without purpose or meaning. Therefore, it is essential to find ways to fill time that contributes to quality of life by providing opportunities for meaningful engagement.

Music is one use of time that improves the quality of life by providing meaningful and purposeful activities that are accessible, are available, can be actively or passively participated in, and can be employed readily by people who are well or people who have illnesses or disabilities. For many older people, music can provide a diversion from unpleasant circumstances, illness, daily stress, and even pain or discomfort. It can give "time out" from the tedium of daily life and contribute quality to life, which is eagerly anticipated.

Music used by individuals for diversion or entertainment can include singing, playing, listening, and even dancing. Setting aside a time each day to sing not only provides a pleasing way to use the time but also provides physical stimulation and subsequent relaxation through deep breathing, expending physical effort, and vocally expressing emotions and feelings. Singing can also include cognitive stimulation, particularly if one studies the history, style, and form of the music used. One may also choose to study vocal production and diction with a professional, but even if one merely sings familiar, favorite songs, singing contributes meaningful, productive experiences to life.

Like singing, playing music on a variety of instruments provides opportunities for pleasurable uses of time. Playing an instrument can reflect and help one to express feelings or simply provide a satisfying experience. Physical stimulation is integral to playing music, and cognitive stimulation, which helps to maintain alertness, interest, and general intellection function, can also be a component. Instrumental playing using percussion instruments is successful merely by maintaining the pulse of a rhythmic beat. Such playing involves little, if any, cognitive processing and is therefore accessible even to those who have severe cognitive losses.

Listening to 20–30 minutes of music once or twice a day requires little effort or skill, and it provides opportunities for rest from work or other activity and diversion from inactivity. While listening, one may sing along with certain song, tap a foot or a knee in rhythm with the music, or play an instrumental accompaniment. For further cognitive stimulation, one may choose to study the musical form, origin, history, and venues for performance as well as listen to a number of renditions of a particular piece of music and delineate the characteristics of each.

Dancing stimulates physical responses and increases heart rate, respiration, and blood pressure. People who dance say it makes them feel better, lifts their spirits, and helps them forget their aches and pains. When performed with a partner, dancing also provides an opportunity to be held in someone's arms. Physical touch may be the most important factor in a satisfying dance experience, but even when performed solo, dance can contribute to physical endurance and flexibility.

Other diversional participation with music may include exercising and background music in order to relieve boredom and enhance endurance. Music videos provide another enjoyable and constructive use of time. These are readily available through video rental resources or are free when borrowed from the local public library. These videos may be videotapes of Broadway musicals, movies that feature song and dance numbers, or musical television programs.

Although music can provide constructive, meaningful uses of time, it can lose its effectiveness if used continuously. With the constant use of music, individuals become attenuated and lose interest. If the use of music is interrupted periodically throughout the day with silence or other activities, the music maintains its effectiveness in focusing attention, providing sensory stimulation, offering diversion from routines, and providing meaningful uses of time.

Outside the home, people may experience music by attending concerts or other musical productions in the community. They may go to free piano, dance, or other recitals offered by teachers and their students, where a receptive audience is appreciated. They may attend musical presentations at the local public library, school or university, senior center, church, synagogue, or other community facility. They may attend dances at their community centers. They may also participate in tours to places that have a focus on musical shows or productions, such as New York City. They may even join a group of people who are interested in making music together regularly. This group may be a chorus or an instrumental ensemble of some type that occasionally performs in the community. Along with performance and regular practice in such groups, it is also possible to share musical skills by teaching people of all ages, by accompanying another musician or group of musicians, and by mentoring and supporting others in their efforts to participate in music.

Another alternative for using free time meaningfully is to engage in the study of music history. This may involve the study of a particular time period, a musical instrument and its development, or the evolution of certain musical forms, such as opera, marching band music, or music used in films or commercial television. One may study ethnic music or, coupled with genealogical research, the music of the times. One may also compose music that serves as a sort of record of family history. Whether or not the music can be notated, this music can be recorded on audio- or videotape and played for many years and generations to come.

One important way to include music as a productive way to use leisure time is to learn a new musical skill or to relearn an old one. Gibbons (1982) showed that older people retain their musical abilities and can learn new skills. She also demonstrated the success with which people in their 70s and 80s can learn or relearn to play musical instruments (Gibbons, 1984). With a good instructor, older people can learn the music they have always wanted to sing or play but did not have the time or opportunity to do so. Considerations must be made for any physical limitations that may impede success, such as arthritic fingers that prohibit or severely limit one's ability to hold an instrument while playing. Adaptive devices can aid success, provided they are designed to accommodate an individual's particular needs.

In addition to physical limitations to holding musical instruments, instruments that require blowing can have deleterious effects on physical health and well-being. This may occur because wind or brass instruments have air resistance, which requires a person to use breath support and air pressure in order to make sounds. Blowing against air resistance tends to increase blood pressure, which can be harmful for people with hypertension. At the same time, blowing against air resistance may build vital capacity and thus may have healthful effects in other people. The breath support sufficient to play a wind instrument also requires abdominal muscle control, which may be contraindicated for people with some physical conditions, such as hernias. Embouchure (lips, mouth, tongue, teeth, and jaw placements), which involves facial muscle tension, may affect other conditions. It is essential, then, to consult a physician concerning specific physical activities associated with playing musical instruments that might affect health and well-being.

Music as an Effective Therapeutic Medium

Music Is Flexible
Other than pervasiveness, one of the most important charac-

teristics that makes music viable as a therapeutic medium is its flexibility. Music has the capacity to be simple or complex, to match a broad spectrum of moods and emotions, to complement diverse social and cultural contexts, to facilitate interaction, to draw people together in cooperation, and to tap residual skills and abilities. This flexibility allows the music therapist to adapt the music to meet an individual client's physical, psychological, and social needs. This adaptability allows for successful experiences, even when people are severely dysfunctional.

The success of participating in music therapy can be defined in a variety of ways, depending upon the skills and ability of the individual for whom it was designed. These successful experiences can range from sitting quietly in a chair to imitating a rhythm pattern on a drum to playing a piano solo. For some people, success is defined as staying in the room while music therapy is conducted; for others, success may be singing a verse of a song.

In order to design music therapy applications that promote success, it is essential to have some knowledge of each client's skills and abilities. Initial and ongoing assessments of these skills and abilities are obtained throughout treatment. Combined with information collected from professionals in other disciplines, such as physical therapy, speech therapy, occupational therapy, and medicine, music therapy assessment outcomes are used to develop goal-directed programs for individual clients. Also important in this process is knowledge of the abilities of individual clients to perform activities of daily living and the functions of daily living, the client's desires for treatment outcomes, and the family's needs for providing and managing care.

Music Is Structured and Occurs Through Time

The therapeutic benefits of music therapy depend largely on the structure and order that is inherent in it (Sears, 1968). Music is structured and thus predictable. It is predictable whether or not it is familiar, because it has rhythm and one beat always follows the next. When the music is familiar, the rhythm and other musical elements, such as melody, harmony, texture, timbre, form, and dynamics, occur in predictable patterns. This predictability in musical elements is comforting and reassuring, at least for the duration.

The only way music can be perceived is through time, and that perception, coupled with predictability, provides a structural framework for time. This time structure provides organization and order. In music therapy interventions, the structure provided by music is used to achieve a range of therapeutic benefits, including anxiety control and stress management, self-control, and social integration.

Music therapy is effective in relieving anxiety and stress because the structure of the music and the order it provides allow for feelings of security. This security is compatible with feelings associated with anxiety and stress (e.g., uneasiness, apprehension, fear). As people choose to allow music to provide security and comfort through its structure, they can let go of deleterious feelings and experience relief, at least for the duration of the music. With practice it is possible for some people to associate feelings of comfort and security with a particular piece of music. Upon hearing the music, they can summon comfort. For some people who have a great deal of experience, comfort can be obtained merely by thinking of the music.

Music may also be used in a therapeutic setting to structure experiences that elicit behaviors that require self-control and responsibility, the prerequisites to social integration with others. These self-managed behaviors are evident in individuals' observable participation in music. People may tap their toes, sing, or play an instrument, which indicates overtly their involvement, commitment, and ability to control and direct their participation. Duration and frequency of participation can be observed and measured. Through such measurement, it can be determined whether the individual has changed behaviors over time; if the person has changed behaviors, the direction and degree of the change can be assessed. Participation can be judged also for its appropriateness within a particular context. When participation is either inadequate or inappropriate for a person's abilities, music therapy interventions can be altered in an effort to better accommodate the person's needs.

Appropriate participation within the structure of music leads to opportunities for cooperation and participation with others. These opportunities are often rare for people who are isolated because of disease processes or other factors that limit their abilities to initiate or respond in most social interactions. Their need to belong with others, to have a sense of community, and to feel the comfort of being an integral member of a group of people has not diminished, but the means to meet these needs may have been lost. Through the use of a music therapy intervention designed to suit individual ability levels, each person can function successfully, either making music or responding to it. When individuals are gathered together to actively participate in music, they have an awareness of being together that develops over time into belonging together. This awareness may also be experienced by persons who have dementia and have lost abilities to relate socially in other ways. The structured, secure, and predictable participation in music provided by the music therapist affords relief from isolation and the loneliness that may be associated with it.

Music is one art form that is accessible to most people. It is available in the environment daily, and opportunities to participate in musical events or performances abound. Because of the accessibility, most people have some sort of personal history with music, and they enjoy their experiences with it. Consequently, music attracts individuals who seek to increase their positive experiences, and it is this attraction that facilitates their involvement in using music therapeutically. People are more likely to enter into a therapeutic intervention and make a commitment to it when it employs a medium, such as music, that facilitates positive experiences.

Music Is Viable in Therapeutic Interventions

The success of music therapy has a lengthy history, much of which is included in the research literature that demonstrates the effects of music on people of all ages. Yet much is unknown about the influence of music on behavior. What is certain is that most people respond to music in some way, and the most efficacious uses of music to influence these responses must be carefully and individually designed. This music must be implemented with continuous observations of behavioral outcomes, ongoing assessments of these outcomes, and the evaluation of changes in individual responses.

Research with older people has indicated that music may be used therapeutically to enhance physical rehabilitation in people who have had strokes (Thaut et al., 1992, 1993; Thaut, McIntosh, & Rice, 1997) and persons diagnosed with Parkinson's disease (McIntosh, Thaut, Rice, Miller, Rathbun, & Brault, 1995; Miller, Thaut, McIntosh & Rice, 1996; Thaut, McIntosh, Rice, Miller, Rathbun, & Brault,

1996). The use of music also enhances the exercise regimens of frail older people and older people (Johnson, Otto, & Clair, 2001; Terasaki, 1993). This implies that music can facilitate enjoyment during exercise programs and may subsequently facilitate adherence to the programs. It is well established that music can facilitate social integration for older, physically frail people (Palmer, 1977), well older people (Gibbons, 1984), and people with Alzheimer's disease or dementia (Brotons & Marti, 2003; Clair, 1991a, 1991b, 1996; Clair & Bernstein, 1990a, 1990b; Clair, Bernstein, & Johnson, 1995; Clair & Ebberts, 1997; Clair & Hanser, 1995) and their spouses (Clair, 2002b; Clair & Hanser, 1995; Clair, Tebb, & Bernstein, 1993). Music therapy also contributes to physical comfort during surgery (Bally, Campbell, Chesnick, & Tranmer, 2003; Spingte, 1989; Standley, 1986, 1992) and other invasive medical procedures (Malone, 1996; Metzler & Berman, 1991; Noguchi, 2006; Presner, Yowler, Smith, Steele, & Fratianne, 2001). Clinical practice demonstrates that music therapy further contributes to the quality of life of older people by providing relief from stress and diversion from ongoing conditions or circumstances and by offering opportunities for meaningful experiences.

Although it is often expected that music will have positive effects on people, it is possible for music to cause damage; for example, the music that positively affects one person may have a deleterious effect on another person. This is illustrated by health care providers who listen to music they enjoy as they perform duties in residential care homes. The health care providers use music that stimulates them as they perform routine care tasks, such as bathing, dressing, repositioning, or feeding a resident; cleaning the resident's room; or changing bed linens with the resident present. The care providers may not notice the effects that the music has on the residents, who may respond with agitated movements and vocalizations that may escalate into screaming, stubbornness, or withdrawal from engagement. In the most extreme circumstances, these residents may become physically combative and require medications to manage their behaviors. With the use of music designed to facilitate relaxation and calm, residents' behaviors could be more cooperative, or at least noncombative, but health care providers would need to manage their decreased energy levels. Perhaps health care tasks that involve residents could be alternated with tasks that do not, allowing the caregivers some task performance time at higher energy levels away from residents that is facilitated by music of their choice.

Like the differences in musical preferences between health care workers and residents in care facilities, music preferences among older people vary markedly. Some individuals may prefer to listen to religious music, but the same music may elicit angry responses or feelings or grief in other people. Some people may prefer only country music played at high volume, whereas others may find the same music tasteless and even offensive.

Although differences in musical preferences may lead to negative reactions, stimulative and sedative music may also elicit mixed responses (Clair & Bernstein, 1994). Some people may respond to certain stimulative music by becoming agitated, noncooperative, and disengaged, whereas others may respond to the same music with increased alert behaviors, as indicated by head turns to locate sights and sounds, eye contact, pleasant facial expressions, more erect posture, better eating patterns, increased pulse rate, and more rapid respirations. These individuals may require stimulative music to emerge from a lethargic, nonresponsive state. Quiet, calming music, then, may have negative effects on these people by promoting and maintaining their inactivity, unless the music is used to quiet them just prior to sleep.

CONCLUSION

Although music has diverse effects on behavior, the effectiveness of certain music for specific purposes must be demonstrated by a qualified professional music therapist. That demonstration will indicate the outcomes of that particular application with that particular person at that point in time. In the event results are not forthcoming or are not those expected, the trained music therapist can alter the approach until a desirable outcome is achieved. With the music therapist's expert knowledge, skill, and ability, the use of music for specific outcomes with individuals can be the most effective and therefore the most viable.

REFERENCES

American Music Therapy Association. (2006a). Certification board for music therapists. In *The 2006 AMTA member sourcebook* (p. xi). Silver Spring, MD: Author.

American Music Therapy Association. (2006b). Standards of clinical practice. In *The 2006 AMTA member sourcebook* (p. 19). Silver Spring, MD: Author.

American Music Therapy Association. (2007). *Music therapy and Alzheimer's disease.* Retrieved from http://www.musictherapy.org/factsheets.html

Bally, K., Campbell, D., Chesnick, K., & Tranmer, J. E. (2003). Effects of patient controlled music therapy during coronary angiography on procedural pain and anxiety distress syndrome. *Critical Care Nurse*, 23(2), 50–57.

Boxberger, R. (1963). *A historical study of the National Association for Music Therapy*. Unpublished doctoral dissertation, University of Kansas, Lawrence.

Brocklesby, R. (1749). *Reflections on the power of music*. London: M. Cooper.

Brotons, M., & Marti, P. (2003). Music therapy with Alzheimer's patients and their families: A pilot project. *Journal of Music Therapy*, 40(2), 138–150.

Bruscia, K. E. (1998). *Defining music therapy* (2nd ed.). Gilsum, NH: Barcelona.

Cevasco, A. M., & Grant, R. E. (2006). Value of musical instruments used by the therapist to elicit responses from individuals in various stages of Alzheimer's disease. *Journal of Music Therapy*, 43(3), 226–246.

Clair, A. A. (1991a). Music therapy for a severely regressed person with probable diagnosis of Alzheimer's disease: A case study. In K. Bruscia (Ed.), *Case studies in music therapy* (pp. 571–580). Phoenixville, PA: Barcelona.

Clair, A. A. (1991b). Rhythmic responses in elderly and their implications for music therapy practice. *Journal of the International Association of Music for the Handicapped*, 6(1), 3–11.

Clair, A. A. (1994). Ethics and values in music therapy for persons who are elderly. In P. Villani (Ed.), *Ethics and values in long term health care* (pp. 27–46). New York: Haworth Press.

Clair, A. A. (1996). The effects of singing on alert responses in persons with late-stage dementia. *Journal of Music Therapy*, 33(4), 234–247.

Clair, A. A. (2002a). Dance for emotional intimacy: Simple one-to-one interventions for family caregivers with loved ones in late-stage dementia. *The Activities Directors' Quarterly for Alzheimer's and Other Dementia Patients*, 3(1), 33–41.

Clair, A. A. (2002b). The effect of caregiver implemented music applications on mutual engagement in caregiver and care receiver couples with dementia. *The American Journal of Alzheimer's Disease & Other Dementias*, 17(5), 286–290.

Clair, A. A. (2002c). Practical ways to use music to manage agitated behaviors in late stage dementia. *The Activities Directors' Quarterly for Alzheimer's and Other Dementia Patients*, 3(1), 41–48.

Clair, A. A., & Bernstein, B. (1990a). A comparison of singing, vibrotactile and nonvibrotactile instrumental playing responses in severely regressed persons with dementia of the Alzheimer's type. *Journal of Music Therapy*, 27(3), 199–125.

Clair, A. A., & Bernstein, B. (1990b). A preliminary study of music therapy programming for severely regressed persons with Alzheimer's type dementia. *Journal of Applied Gerontology*, 9(3), 299–311.

Clair, A. A., & Bernstein, B. (1994). The effect of no music, stimulative music and sedative music on agitated behaviors in persons with severe dementia. *Activities, Adaptations, and Aging*, 19(1), 61–70.

Clair, A. A., Bernstein, B., & Johnson, G. (1995). Rhythmic characteristics in persons diagnosed with dementia, including those with probable Alzheimer's type. *Journal of Music Therapy*, 32(2), 113–131.

Clair, A. A., & Ebberts, A. (1997). The effects of music therapy on interactions between family caregivers and their care receivers with late stage dementia. *Journal of Music Therapy*, 34(3), 148–164.

Clair, A. A., & Hanser, S. (1995). Music therapy: Retrieving the losses of dementia of the Alzheimer's type for patient and caregiver. In T. Wigram, R. West, & B. Saperston (Eds.), *The art and science of music therapy: A handbook* (pp. 342–360). Chur, Switzerland: Harwood Academic.

Clair, A. A., & O'Konski, M. (2006). The effect of Rhythmic Auditory Stimulation (RAS) on gait characteristics of cadence, velocity, and stride length in persons with late stage dementia. *Journal of Music Therapy*, 43(2), 154–163.

Clair, A. A., Tebb, S., & Bernstein, B. (1993, January/February). The effects of a socialization and music therapy intervention on self-esteem and loneliness in spouse caregivers of those diagnosed with dementia of the Alzheimer's type: A pilot study. *American Journal of Alzheimer's Care and Related Disorders and Research*, 24–32.

Daly, J. (2005). *Evidence-based medicine and the search for a science of clinical care.* Berkeley: University of California Press.

Davis, W. (1987). Music therapy in 19th century America. *Journal of Music Therapy*, 24(2), 76–87.

Davis, W. (1993). Keeping the dream alive: Profiles of three early twentieth century music therapists. *Journal of Music Therapy*, 30(1), 34–45.

Davis, W. B., & Gfeller, K. E. (1999). Music therapy: An historical perspective. In W. B. Davis, K. E. Gfeller, & M. H. Thaut (Eds.), *An introduction to music therapy theory and practice* (2nd ed.) (pp. 17–37). Dubuque, IA: Wm. C. Brown.

Flowers, P. J., & Murphy, J. W. (2001). Talking about music: Interviews with older adults about their music education, preferences, activities, and reflections. Update: *Applications of Research in Music Education*, 20(1), 26–32.

Forever young–Music and aging: Hearing before the Senate Special Committee on Aging, 102nd Cong., 1st Sess. (1991).

Gaston, E. T. (1968). Man and music. In E. T. Gaston (Ed.), *Music in therapy* (pp. 7–29). New York: Macmillan.

Gfeller, K. (2002a). Music as communication. In M. H. Thaut & R. G. Unkefer (Eds.), *Music therapy in the treatment of adults with mental disorders: Theoretical bases and clinical interventions* (pp. 42–59). St. Louis, MO: MMB Music.

Gfeller, K. (2002b). Music as a therapeutic agent: Historical and sociocultural perspectives. In M. H. Thaut & R. G. Unkefer (Eds.), *Music therapy in the treatment of adults with mental disorders: Theoretical bases and clinical interventions* (pp. 60–67). St. Louis, MO: MMB Music.

Gfeller, K. (2002c). The function of aesthetic stimuli in the therapeutic process. In M. H. Thaut & R. G. Unkefer (Eds.), *Music* therapy in the treatment of adults with mental disorders: Theoretical bases and clinical interventions (pp. 68–85). St. Louis, MO: MMB Music.

Gibbons, A. C. (1977). Pop musical preferences of elderly persons. Journal of Music Therapy, 14(4), 180–189.

Gibbons, A. C. (1982). Musical Aptitude Profile scores in a non-institutionalized elderly population. Journal of Research in Music Education, 30(1), 23–29.

Gibbons, A. C. (1984). A program for non-institutionalized, mature adults: A description. Activities, Adaptations, and Aging, 6(1), 71–80.

Gibbons, A. C., & Heller, G. N. (1985). Music therapy in Handel's England. College Music Symposium, 25(1), 59–72.

Groene, R. (2001). The effect of presentation and accompaniment styles on attentional and responsive behaviors of participants with dementia diagnoses. Journal of Music Therapy, 38(1), 36–50.

Hamburg, J., & Clair, A. A. (2003). The effects of a movement with music program on measures of balance and gait speed in healthy older adults. Journal of Music Therapy, 40(3), 212–226.

Heller, G. (1987). Ideas, initiatives, and implementations: Music therapy in America, 1789–1848. Journal of Music Therapy, 24(1), 35–46.

Hodges, D. A. (1980). Handbook of music psychology. Silver Spring, MD: National Association for Music Therapy.

Johnson, G., Otto, D., & Clair, A. A. (2001). The effect of instrumental and vocal music on adherence to a physical rehabilitation exercise program with persons who are elderly. Journal of Music Therapy, 38(2), 82–96.

Jonas, J. L. (1991). Preferences of elderly music listeners residing in nursing homes for art music, traditional jazz, popular music of today, and country music. *Journal of Music Therapy*, 23(3), 149–160.

Lathom, M., Peterson, M., & Havlicek, L. (1982). Musical preferences of older people attending nutrition sites. *Educational Gerontology*, 8(2), 155–165.

Malone, A. B. (1996). The effects of live music on the distress of pediatric patients receiving intravenous starts, venipunctures, injections, and heel sticks. *Journal of Music Therapy*, 23(1), 19–33.

McIntosh, G., Thaut, M., Rice, R., Miller, R., Rathbun, J., & Brault, J. (1995). Rhythmic facilitation in gait training of Parkinson's disease. *Annals of Neurology*, 38(2), 331.

Merriam, A. P. (1964). *The anthropology of music*. Evanston, IL: Northwestern University Press.

Metzler, R., & Berman, T. (1991). The effects of sedative music on the anxiety of bronchoscopy patients. In C. D. Maranto (Ed.), *Applications of music in medicine* (pp. 163–178). Silver Spring, MD: National Association for Music Therapy.

Miller, R., Thaut, M., McIntosh, G., & Rice, R. (1996). Components of EMG variability in Parkinsonian and healthy elderly gait. *Electroencephalography and Clinical Neurophysiology*, 101(1), 1–7.

Nettl, B. (1956). *Music in primitive cultures*. Cambridge, MA: Harvard University Press.

Noguchi, L. K. (2006). The effect of music versus nonmusic on behavioral signs of distress and self-report of pain in pediatric injection patients. *Journal of Music Therapy*, 43(1), 16–38.

Palmer, M. (1977). Music therapy in a comprehensive program of treatment and rehabilitation for the geriatric resident. *Journal of Music Therapy*, 14(4), 190–197.

Presner, J. D., Yowler, C. J., Smith, L. F., Steele, A. L., & Fratianne, R. B. (2001). Music therapy for assistance with pain and anxiety management in burn treatment. *Journal of Burn Care and Rehabilitation*, 22(1), 83–88.

Radocy, R., & Boyle, J. D. (2003). *Psychological foundations of musical behavior* (4th ed.). Springfield, IL: Charles C. Thomas.

Roskam, K. S. (1993). *Feeling the sound: The influence of music on behavior*. San Francisco: San Francisco Press.

Sears, W. (1968). Processes in music therapy. In E. T. Gaston (Ed.), *Music in therapy* (pp. 30–44). New York: Macmillan.

Shapiro, D. W., Laskerk R. D., Bindman, A. B., & Lee, P. R. (1993). Containing costs while improving quality of care: The role of profiling and practice guideline. *Annual Review of Public Health*, 14, 219–241.

Spingte, R. (1989). The anxiolytic effects of music. In M. Lee (Ed.), *Rehabilitation, music and human well-being* (pp. 82–97). St. Louis, MO: MMB Music.

Standley, J. (1986). Music research in medical/dental treatment: Meta-analysis and clinical applications. *Journal of Music Therapy*, 23(2), 56–122.

Standley, J. (1992). Meta-analysis of research in music and medical treatment: Effect size as a basis for comparison across multiple dependent and independent variables. In R. Spintge & R. Droh (Eds.), *Music medicine* (pp. 364–378). St. Louis, MO: MMB Music.

Terasaki, Y. (1993). *The effect of music and exercise on elbow exten-*

sion and flexion in elderly care home residents. Unpublished master's thesis, The University of Kansas, Lawrence.

Thaut, M. (2002). Neuropsychological processes in music perception and their relevance in music therapy. In M. H. Thaut & R. G. Unkefer (Eds.), *Music therapy in the treatment of adults with mental disorders: Theoretical bases and clinical interventions* (pp. 2–32). St. Louis, MO: MMB Music.

Thaut, M., McIntosh, G., Prassas, S., & Rice, R. (1992). Effect of auditory rhythmic pacing on normal gait and gait in stroke, cerebellar disorder, and transverse myelitis. In M. Woollacott & E. Horak (Eds.), *Posture and gait: Control mechanisms* (pp. 437–440). Eugene, OR: University of Oregon Books.

Thaut, M., McIntosh, G., Prassas, S., & Rice, R. (1993). The effect of auditory rhythmic cueing on stride and EMG patterns in hemiparetic gait of stroke patients. *Journal of Neurologic Rehabilitation*, 7(1), 9–16.

Thaut, M. H., McIntosh, G. C., & Rice, R. R. (1997). Rhythmic facilitation of gait training in hemiparetic stroke rehabilitation. *Journal of the Neurological Sciences*, 151(2), 207–212.

Thaut, M., McIntosh, G., Rice, R., Miller, R., Rathbun, J., & Brault, J. (1996). Rhythmic auditory stimulation in gait training for Parkinson's disease patients. *Movement Disorders*, 11(2), 193–200.

United States National Library of Medicine, National Institutes of Health. (2004). *Outcomes Core Library Recommendations, 2004.* Retrieved January 7, 2007, from http://www.nlm.nih.gov/nichsr/corelib/houtcomes.html

Whitehead-Pleaux, A. M., Baryza, M. J., & Sheridan, R. L. (2006). The effects of music therapy on pediatric patients' pain and anxiety during donor site dressing change. *Journal of Music Therapy*, 43(2), 136–153.

Chapter 2

Therapeutic Music for Healthy Older Adults

Therapeutic Music for Healthy Older Adults

Traditionally wellness has been defined as an absence of disease, but more recent considerations of wellness also include a positive approach to staying healthy and becoming healthier (Bolton, 1985). With positive approaches to wellness, many components are added. These include those that relate to physical, social, and psychological well-being, with a focus on the prevention of disease rather than on the cure. Wellness has become the development of a lifestyle that promotes the best possible health (Bolton, 1985). Health and wellness no longer refer merely to an absence of diagnosis but to developing and maintaining the best possible function, even with one or more diagnoses (World Health Organization, 2001).

Evidence is strong that social activity, personal control, and opportunities to increase knowledge and skills contribute to a sense of well-being in older people (Feldman & Oberlink, 2003; Greenfield & Marks, 2007; Okun, Olding, & Cohn, 1990) and subsequently to their wellness. Therefore, activities are recommended that (1) promote social interactions with others, (2) offer opportunities to make decisions and manage choices, (3) present occasions to learn or relearn information or skills, and (4) provide opportunities to discover novel ways to use personal resources. Participation in music involves all of these and more.

MUSIC AND WELLNESS

Perhaps one of the best ways to be well is to remain interested in life and to participate as fully as possible in it. The mode of participation must be left to individual choice, and that choice may be influenced by physical, cognitive, and social abilities and opportunities. Music can be central to that which stimulates interest and motivates participation.

Involvement in music throughout life is becoming important to people and to music merchants. These merchants know that music is a source of great satisfaction, and they are beginning to understand its appeal to older people. Keyboard programs for older beginners are available and include materials for learning that are designed to facilitate success. Gone are the days when a music company sold chord organs and provided customers with a color-coded music book with which to learn at home on their own. Music companies now offer instructions to support individuals in active music making, whatever their musical instrument.

Learning music and participating in it appeals to older people who value wellness and prevention of disease, because involvement with music promotes physical and psychological well-being (Koga, 2005; VanWeelden & Whipple, 2004). When people have success with music, feelings of accomplishment and satisfaction dominate feelings of pain and discomfort. Efforts are directed toward personal productivity and pleasurable results. Boredom is relieved, and people are motivated to maintain their levels of functioning in order to continue the rewarding activities. Subsequently, people experience positive emotional responses. They report that generally they "feel good."

People who tend to focus only on their aches and pains tend to feel progressively more discomfort; as they do, they lose their motivation to involve themselves in activities. They feel "too bad" to go anywhere or to do anything. They are understimulated and often bored. They may experience feelings of depression as they think only of their poor health and their unsatisfactory lifestyles. With lack of motivation, they become sedentary and progressively more debilitated.

> Mr. Simmons, age 82, was an exemplar of well-being as he participated in a music program for healthy older adults. Although he had arthritis in his hands and fingers, which gave him constant pain, he was determined to remain active. He involved himself in activities that motivated him to leave his easy chair, and he practiced playing the piano every day. He said that every time he began to play, his fingers felt stiff and painful, but as he forced himself to play, his fingers became more limber and hurt less. He said that he dreaded sitting down at the keyboard, but he liked the music so much that he wanted to play. He knew each time that his hands and fingers would eventually feel somewhat better if he just continued to play. This man also said that he was quite aware that if he stopped playing for any length of time, his fingers would stiffen so that he could not use them at all. Therefore, he used piano playing as a motivator for finger dexterity exercises, which added to his enjoyment as they maintained his physical function.

Other people involved in daily physical exercise programs to maintain their strength and flexibility have found the exercises tedious. Although they do not actually enjoy the exercises, they enjoy the healthy feelings that result from doing them regularly. However, motivation is sometimes a problem. Using music helps these people remain committed to their exercise programs. A woman who incorporated music into her walking program commented, "You know, I used to dread my morning walks, but now I just put on my headset and go. I think nothing of it listening to my favorite music, and you know, it seems I am finished with my three miles in a fraction of the time."

Music has become a great motivator to exercise for many older people (Bernard, 1992; Johnson, Otto, & Clair, 2001) including those who have late stage dementia (Mathews, Clair, & Kosloski, 2001). The tempo and rhythm of the music maintain their rhythmic participation and help to increase their endurance. By using music, they find the exercise more pleasant, they are amazed at how quickly the time seems to pass, and they find they can tolerate exercising regularly.

DEVELOPMENT OF MUSICAL SKILLS

Many healthy older people have the time and energy to pursue a host of interests, including music. Some older people have long desired to develop musical skills, such as learning to play an instrument, learning to sing, or relearning a musical skill acquired earlier. Other older people have been musically active all their lives by teaching and/or performing. Regardless of the age at which people begin their musical experiences, music provides great potential for enhanced quality of life and subsequent wellness (Coffman, 2002).

Traditionally, people begin their music education in elementary school. Programs that introduce instrumental study are generally targeted toward a particular grade level. If people do not have the inclination or the opportunity to begin music at that given entry point, they are generally unlikely to do so later in life. They may pursue private music study as adults, but most people are discouraged by the mistaken belief that music study should begin in childhood, if music development and learning are expected (Bowles, 1991; Jellison, 1999). Success is possible for some people who, in frustration, gave up early attempts to learn music. For example, a woman who had failed to learn to play the piano when she was a child decided to take lessons in her 60s. Her account of her experiences as a nontraditional student revealed the following:

1. The skills she had learned previously came back quickly.

2. Music she played brought memories of events and positive feelings that she experienced years before.

3. Making music presented opportunities to interact socially with others, including people she had not seen in years.

4. The enjoyment she received from playing the piano was so great that time seemed to pass without notice.

5. Her playing success motivated continued efforts to practice (Adams, 1995).

The capacity to learn music remains viable throughout life, and research indicates clearly that older people retain their musical abilities (Bruhn, 2002). Furthermore, these abilities remain strong through the ninth decade and beyond, whether people live independently or in residential care (Gibbons, 1982a, 1983).

People who have musical ability have the capacity to relearn music or to develop musical skills for the first time, even if they are older. The potential for older adults to successfully learn and perform music in their 70s and 80s was demonstrated by Clair, who published under the name of Gibbons (1984) a description of an innovative program. The goals of the program were to teach university music therapy students how to design and implement appropriate learning experiences with nontraditional, older pupils, and to provide older adults with opportunities to learn musical skills. The older people in the program were either studying music for the first time or had learned musical skills earlier in their lives but had not used them for several decades. One of the students had been a flute major in college but had not played the instrument for 50 years. These older people met either in small groups or individually with a college-age tutor for 1 hour each week, and they gathered as a group to participate in music for a 1½-hour session conducted by a music therapist at the conclusion of each week. All music materials were adapted and arranged for the participants, who played an assortment of instruments, including guitar, autoharp, flute, clarinet, harmonica, electric vibraphone, piano, and trap set drums. In addition, the group included an array of singers. During most weeks, 20–25 people participated in the program.

Music was designed to meet the musical skill level of each older student and was previewed in the tutoring sessions to promote sufficient skill development for eventual success in the group. For instance, new guitar players learned songs in their tutoring sessions, and when their skills were sufficient, the songs were added to the group's repertoire. The tutors helped guitar-playing participants move their fingers for chord changes and hear and see in the musical notation the points at which chord changes occurred in the songs. The flutist and other players were given parts adapted for skills that ranged from playing melodies to playing harmonies. Regardless of the musical instrument used, including the voice, the older people were encouraged to practice, which they did regularly and productively.

The outcome of the program was an ensemble that met each week. The weekly rehearsals were so successful that participants were eager to share their musical performances with others. They often volunteered to perform at local residential care facilities and for church and civic programs in the community. They were also featured performers at two statewide Governor's Conferences on Aging.

Participants in the program reached their desired goals, and some of them became proficient. They expressed dissatisfaction with mediocre musical products and consistently strove to achieve the best performances possible (Gibbons, 1982b). When desired musical goals were met, the participants were eager to perform. The following examples demonstrate their eagerness:

> For everyone who asked, Mrs. Asher demonstrated her new abilities to play guitar accompaniment while she sang her favorite songs. Her family was so impressed by her musical accomplishments that they gave her a new guitar for her 82nd birthday. The same family members had laughed at her 8 months earlier when she had announced, "I'm going to take up the guitar 'cause I've always wanted to play one and now there's time to practice." Mrs. Asher developed skill suffi-

cient to play all of her favorite songs and sang them to others, especially to her friends who were in residential care facilities.

Mrs. Taub, who had studied flute as a music major in college, began after approximately 1 year in the group to play some of her college repertoire. She developed sufficient breath control and fingering dexterity to play duets at church services with a younger man who taught flute at the local university. Mrs. Taub also confidently played solos for all types of audiences. She said, "Playing my flute has been like learning to ride a bicycle. With a little practice, it all came back!"

Members of the music program were given choices concerning their mode of learning music (e.g., note reading, playing by rote). Although the flute soloist wanted to relearn the skills to read and play complex music, most people opted for rote learning. However, all participants responded to efforts designed to develop independence in skill development. For instrumentalists, this included learning some basic music theory so that they could determine when certain harmonizations were appropriate. Guitar and piano players, in particular, learned which chords to use in specific keys and learned to determine when a chord was correct within the context of a song. Flute players wrote their own notations, and the drummer worked out a system that he used to remind himself how and where to play certain riffs. Singers learned to use markings for dynamic changes and developed some of their own written cues. All skills were taught in an effort to reduce dependence upon the music therapist who facilitated the group and to foster independence and self-reliance so that people could attempt to play and sing on their own at home and in other contexts.

Social Integration Through Musical Skill Development

When a commitment is made to accept responsibility for performing one's musical part and to contribute to the success of others, camaraderie develops among the participants. Musical experiences subsequently contribute to a sense of community in which people share concern for each other. They are attentive to each other as they respond to others' personal needs to share times of joy, sadness, fear, or grief. The following example illustrates this well:

> Miss Camden, who participated regularly in the music therapy clinical program for older adults, was diagnosed with cancer. She told her fellow musicians that she was about to undergo treatment that would keep her away from rehearsals for a time. Group members took turns visiting her in the hospital after her surgery and at home during recuperation and follow-up chemotherapy. The group rallied to lend support to one of their own and to offer comfort at a time of distress. When Miss Camden was well enough to return to the group, they welcomed her with enthusiasm. She told them that she was motivated to work on her recovery so that she could participate in music with them again.

As musicians develop camaraderie, they must also develop a working relationship that requires compromise. In the music therapy clinical program, compromise was required in making all decisions, including song selections, performance formats, and performance schedules. Program participants were encouraged to perform as soloists and as members of duets or trios. Materials for and approaches to these performances were structured by the music therapist in order to ensure success. Nonetheless, all group members were required to involve themselves in decision making, which encouraged their expressions of personal preferences and their social interactions. The implementation of their decisions served to develop their self-confidence and their respect for one another.

Thoughtfulness and regard for the importance of each individual were essential components of the musicians' group function. Clear behavioral boundaries were set by the group members and supported by the music therapist, and any lack of consideration was quickly checked, as demonstrated by the following example:

> During a session, Mrs. Bjorklund, who had already made suggestions to the group that were implemented, pushed for more personal control of the session activities by insisting that the group perform another of her favorite songs. She

was reminded that she had already made one song choice for the day and that remaining selections would be made by other members of the group. She replied, "If you're not going to sing my song, then I'm just going to pack up my guitar and go." The music therapist said that it would be fine if she left. Mrs. Bjorklund shouted back that she would just go, and the music therapist quietly helped her gather her things and assisted her out the door. She phoned the music therapist later to apologize for being so pushy and asked whether she had been removed from the group. When Mrs. Bjorklund was assured that she was welcome to attend anytime but that consideration of everyone's choices was necessary, she said she would return the following week. Mrs. Bjorklund subsequently became a regular and pleasant attendee of the group sessions. Although her input for decisions was solicited, she never again pushed the limits for exclusive, personal control.

The social outcomes of the music therapy clinical program went beyond the development of camaraderie among the participants. Friendships developed among the people who met each week. Some of them decided to gather for extra rehearsals outside the tutoring and the large ensemble sessions. These practice sessions sometimes were held several times a week for several hours. Smaller ensembles developed from the additional practice sessions, and the members of these smaller groups grew confident enough to schedule and perform their own programs in the community.

All of the group members enjoyed performing together, and they especially enjoyed working with the university students who were their tutors. Many of them occasionally commented that the "college kids" represented for them their grandchildren. Some of the older people had no grandchildren, and if they did have them, they lived so far away that visits were rare. Although the university students did not think of their older students as their grandparents, they held them in high regard as their elders. Initially, they felt reluctant to give instructions to the older students because they were concerned that they be shown the proper respect. As both tutors and students became acquainted, they established some ground rules for mutual respect. The tutors soon discovered the value of their older students as survivors, people rich in the knowledge gleaned from broad-ranging experiences. These survivors were nonjudgmental, and although they generally did not interfere in their tutors' affairs, they provided comfort and hope when concerns were shared with them. The older adults always had words of encouragement for the young people when they were shaken by changes in their lives, when they were discouraged with schoolwork, or when they suffered disappointments and broken hearts.

The tutors quickly found that the older adults were motivated like no other learners with whom they had worked. The older students practiced consistently and regularly, tried to incorporate every suggestion into their performances, and always came to the tutoring sessions prepared. They never complained about the difficulty of the lessons. Although they sometimes became discouraged with the pace of their progress, the older adults were so eager to learn that they absorbed all they could and then asked for more.

The tutors found their time with their older adult students so personally rewarding that they became even more determined in their efforts to make every learning strategy effective and every tutoring session successful. The older adults responded with undivided attention, diligent work, pleasing accomplishments, and true enjoyment.

The students demonstrated success at some level with every session. Tutors noted these successes as indications of learning and teaching effectiveness, which contributed to everyone's self-confidence and self-esteem. The tutoring sessions and the large ensemble groups were satisfying to both the tutors and the students as a forum for social interaction through musical involvement.

The group of older musicians demonstrated clearly that musical skill development leads to opportunities to use or make music with other people. Through sharing music, people develop mutual concern. The musical ensemble requires all participants to be considerate of one another, to cooperate and compromise, and ultimately to subordinate their individual desires in order to facilitate group success. Therefore, all individuals bring to each group session their particular skills and abilities, which work in tandem to contribute to the success of the whole.

People who do not wish to develop musical skills or who are not musicians can be avid consumers of music. They may gather for mutual enjoyment, either through hearing music performed live or through listening to recordings. Here again, music is the substance that draws these people together in a common interest and engages them socially. They enjoy not only the music, but each other's company as well.

Self-Expression Through Musical Skill Development

In addition to social interaction, the musical skills developed in the music therapy clinical program created opportunities for self-expression for the older adults (Gibbons, 1984). As an example, Mrs. Baeder, a widow who lived alone in an isolated rural area, had learned to play the guitar. When asked how she used her music, she replied:

> I play when I'm happy and joyful because the feelings just come bubbling out, and I feel so glad that I just have to sing and play. I also play when I'm sad and blue and have nowhere else to turn. I think I play guitar pretty well, but I don't think I'm such a good singer. My dog doesn't seem to mind, though. He always comes to lie down at my feet when I get out the guitar. You know, I think he likes it about as much as I do. Anyway, it really makes the hours fly by.

Structuring Time Through Development of Musical Skills

Along with using music to express her feelings, Mrs. Baeder used music to structure the time she spent alone. She described her situation as follows:

> The winter days are the worst. When the snow is deep and I can't get out of the house, the days are so long that they seem to never end. Sometimes I don't see other people for as long as 2 weeks, depending on when the snow plow comes through. I talk on the telephone every day, but that can only last so long. The time goes fastest when I am playing my music.

Other group members participated in music as a way to structure their time. Some older adults spoke of days that were slow because there was so little to do, and others said that they were busier since they retired than when they were working. Participation in music was important to these busy group members, and they worked other activities around it. Whether available time is abundant or scarce, and regardless of active or passive involvement, meaningful musical experiences can serve as the pivotal component in a person's schedule.

Cognitive Stimulation Through Development of Musical Skills

Many people enjoy the cognitive stimulation that music provides. Such stimulation is possible because music is a complex medium that allows room for growth and development and demands some intellectual activity in order to maintain an acquired competency level.

Although the maintenance of skill requires intellectual activity, trying new material brings even greater cognitive challenges, whether one makes or composes music. It is not unusual for older people to meet these challenges through progressively learning more complex or difficult material or through developing more sophisticated skills. For example, Mrs. Baeder, the woman who played guitar in her isolated farmhouse, often asked for new songs and for new techniques in order to play them. She was interested in learning a variety of new strumming and picking patterns, and other than those she was taught, she often developed her own. Whenever she was told that the new material might be difficult at first, she responded, "Honey, I've got the time, I've got the interest, and I have the motivation. Just teach me the songs. I really want to learn."

Self-taught musical skills can also promote cognitive stimulation. Although these skills can take many forms, the following case illustrates one approach:

Mr. Mangoni, age 79, purchased a small electronic keyboard and taught himself to play by ear many songs that were popular during his young adult years. After he had mastered what he called "some respectable renditions of some good old tunes," he decided that he would like to learn to read music. He felt confident enough to attempt to learn on his own and bought a lesson book at the local music store. Mr. Mangoni said that he needed to learn to play the songs in conventional key centers in order to play songs with other people. He had always played his music using only the black piano keys. This type of playing did not transfer well to playing with others who played the same songs in conventional tonalities. Mr. Mangoni was successful in his efforts to teach himself to read music and to play in a number of keys. He said that he enjoyed learning new things and that at his age it was important to stimulate his mind.

Cognitive stimulation using music is not restricted to performing it. Stimulation can also occur through learning about music. People may be particularly interested in music from specific cultures or certain historical periods. They may want to know more about the history of a particular style of music and how it developed. They may want to hear recordings and live renditions of the music as they study its history. Their musical interests may take them to libraries and to other people from whom they may gather information.

Cognitive challenges with music may also be met by composing melodies, lyrics, and/or instrumental parts. These challenges may begin with composing new lyrics for familiar songs. These melodies can be tape recorded until the skill to write musical notation is acquired. Once the music is composed, people can perform it themselves or they can recruit other interested people to perform it.

Whatever skills or abilities one possesses, participating in music contributes to quality of life by bringing great enjoyment, providing relief from boredom, supplying a constructive use of time, and, ultimately, providing an excellent source of expression. The music therapy group for older adult musicians described here was successful in engaging participation among a widely diverse group of older people. Although the description of this program is limited to a group of older adults in a specific community, the potential for other group musical experiences and individual musical skill development is remarkable. Perhaps knowing that other people have achieved their dream to learn music may help to encourage others who have a similar desire. It is important to know that it is never too late to learn to use music to enrich the quality of one's life.

PARTICIPATION IN COMMUNITY MUSIC ACTIVITIES

Individuals can choose to be active participants (performers) or passive participants (consumers) in community music activities. Many older people value the arts and actively support them by purchasing tickets for the symphony, chamber orchestra, and civic chorus. Older adults also lend their support to the younger people in the community by attending school musical productions, even when they do not personally know the participants. Thus, many older people demonstrate a commitment to aesthetic development in their communities through their presence at musical and other artistic events.

In addition to regular attendance at musical performances, older people may contribute to fund-raising efforts for musical productions by soliciting financial commitments from others or by making financial contributions. The time and money they spend to support efforts to make musical events available contribute to their own quality of life and that of their communities.

Older people can also support music in their communities through active music making. Many older adults have musical skills that make them valuable additions to instrumental performing groups of all kinds. Many people who are past retirement age are excellent performers. They can still consistently deliver quality performances. Their many years of experience have seasoned them, and yet they retain freshness and excitement in their mature playing.

Although performing instrumental music in community groups requires many years of study, opportunities may exist for active community participation for older people who enjoy singing but have not had formal training. Community singing groups such as barbershop quartets or other specialized vocal ensembles may serve as valuable resources for people who enjoy singing. Some of these groups restrict their memberships to a certain number and do not add anyone unless someone permanently leaves the group. Some of these groups are further restricted by the audition process, and people who want to join must meet the performance stipulations of the music directors.

Church choirs may be far less limiting because often an effort is made to include all interested individuals. Some drawbacks exist, however. For example, some nonreligious people may not want to sing in association with a religious venue, and some people wish to sing a broader repertoire, one that is not confined to religious music. Singing in some other context is more appropriate for these people.

Perhaps the greatest deterrent to singing for older people is their lack of confidence in their abilities or their lack of comfort with the quality of their voices. This discomfort may result from playing songs in high keys. To enhance success in singing, songs generally must be placed within a singable range, and this range decreases with age (Moore, Staum, & Brotons, 1992).

Older people may also be reluctant to sing because they have had negative experiences with participating in music at some point in their lives. Some may have heard criticisms of other people's singing voices and generalized the comments to themselves. When one woman was asked why she no longer sang although she had always enjoyed singing, she said:

> Why, I wouldn't dare sing because I'm afraid that I sound just terrible. One day a while back, I was walking down the steps of the church after the service and I heard some people behind me comment on the singing they had heard inside. One said, "Did you hear that woman singing off key in front of us? I just couldn't stand it. She really ought to hush up." When I heard those people talking, I thought they might be talking about me. I didn't want to turn around to ask them, so I just decided that I wouldn't sing anymore. I certainly didn't want to make such a racket that it disturbed people in the congregation!

Other people do not sing because they were told, usually at a young age, that their vocal qualities were not pleasing. Others have been told that they could not "carry a tune" and should never sing. The results are heartbreaking:

> A 70-year-old woman, Mrs. Feingold, who was a participant in a music therapy seminar for older people, told the music therapist that she could not sing and that her lack of involvement in the seminar did not mean she was not interested. When asked if she had an injury that prohibited singing, Mrs. Feingold responded, "I was told by a music teacher when I

was a young woman in high school that my voice was so awful that I should never sing. I was so embarrassed. I had no idea that I sounded so bad, but if a music teacher told me, then it must be so." For 50 years Mrs. Feingold had been a passive participant whenever community or church activities involved singing, but when encouraged within the context of the music therapy seminar to vocalize, she began to try. At the close of the 2-day seminar, Mrs. Feingold confessed that she had initially dreaded the musical components of the program, but as she joined the other seminar participants, her singing had brought her great joy. The discouraging comments of one person years before had caused Mrs. Feingold to exclude herself from singing activities. She felt like an outsider, and she expressed regret at missing so much over her lifetime. Follow-up correspondence from Mrs. Feingold indicated that she was continuing to sing every day, although she usually sang when no one was around to listen. She thanked the music therapist for encouraging her to do something that brought her so much enjoyment.

This woman's story is a sad illustration of one of the greatest challenges concerning active participation in music, particularly in older people: the lack of self-confidence and self-worth related to making music. It is essential that people make music for the sheer enjoyment of it and that they realize not all musical outcomes can be or should be perfect. It is also essential for them to know that negative criticism of their music is not a criticism of them. People may misinterpret criticism of their music as a personal rejection. If their musicianship is judged to be inadequate, then they may feel that they too are so judged. Therefore, comments about someone's musical performance must be made in a spirit of goodwill. Unless such commentary is solicited from people who can provide an honest, constructive critique of their performance, they are probably better off not asking for it.

Older People as Dynamic Community Resources

Intergenerational Music Programming in the College Setting

Many older people have remarkable musical skills that can enhance community musical experiences. These people are wonderful community resources, although they are often overlooked unless no one else can provide what is needed. They can be involved as fully contributing members of the community, and failure to include them denies opportunities to people who can benefit from their skill and wastes the gifts these older people have to share. The following example demonstrates how older adults turned a failing orchestra into a thriving performance ensemble:

> A small liberal arts college in the Midwest began including older adult musicians from the community one fall semester when it did not have adequate student enrollment to fill chairs in the college orchestra. Not wanting to disband the orchestra and end a school tradition, the conductor solicited the involvement of musicians of all ages, and people responded graciously. One of the participants was a woman in her late 70s who played violin. She played regularly with other older adults in a string quartet that had been assembled approximately 40 years earlier. She was pleased with playing in a small ensemble but was also eager to participate in an orchestra. She scheduled an audition, performed well, and was urged to join the orchestra as first violin. The twice-weekly rehearsals and seasonal performances presented many more opportunities for her to play, and she contributed significantly to the orchestra by filling a part that would have been impossible without her. Her willingness to join the orchestra not only met her desire to play but also made the orchestra viable.

This small college orchestra became an intergenerational community experience, not only for the audience but also for the players. Traditionally, intergenerational programs are conceived as very old people interacting with very young people, usually preschool-age children. Music makes available many more opportunities for the generations within communities to interact. Consequently, younger people reap the benefits of working with older, more experienced people, and older people have a place of meaning and purpose within their communities. The older people are not forgotten, unproductive members of society. They are viable, vibrant members of the community who contribute something that no one else can give. The following vignette illustrates this concept well:

> Mrs. McIntosh, a pianist, a private piano instructor, and a retired elementary education music teacher, was asked to accompany the local high school chorus when the newly hired choral director requested an accompanist to assist him. Mrs. McIntosh was glad to help. She attended the daily choral rehearsals as the students prepared for the fall concert. She could sight read anything the director put before her and played with great skill. The students responded well to her because it was obvious that she added a great deal to the musicality of their singing.

> The fall concert was a huge success. To Mrs. McIntosh's astonishment, many people in the community complimented her on her playing. They said that she really added to the performance and that they thought it was wonderful that she was willing to work with young people. The choral director was extremely appreciative. He was able to pull off a showy performance that impressed all in attendance. He asked Mrs. McIntosh to continue with him through the spring concert and the spring music contests. She accepted his invitation.

> Mrs. McIntosh began working with the students during school hours and sometimes in the evenings at her home as they prepared for their solos and their small ensemble contest performances. Again, the results of the vocal performances were rewarding for the students, and Mrs. McIntosh was delighted to be a part of it all, from the performances to the school bus rides.

> Mrs. McIntosh is now 78 years old. She continues her work at

the same high level of skill and expertise as when she began 10 years ago. In addition, when the high school students see her in public, they greet her with enthusiasm. It is apparent that they like her very much. On one occasion she commented, "I really don't know why the high school boys, and the girls too, are so friendly. They always stop to talk to me and ask me how I am. It is really odd, don't you think, since I am just an old lady?"

The reason for the students' courtesy is apparent to all who know that the high quality of performance that Mrs. McIntosh is able to inspire is appreciated. She contributes to the success of the students' performances and the increased level of self-esteem that results from success (people who contribute to others' self-esteem are always held in high regard). The students know that they would not give high-quality performances without Mrs. McIntosh's contributions. They acknowledge her skill, which adds satisfaction and excitement to their rehearsals and performances. They think she is "just the greatest!" The choral director is also quick to recognize Mrs. McIntosh's contributions to his success. With her accompaniment, he can count on competent musicianship. He directs with confidence and assurance, knowing that his accompanist will support and enhance the performance.

Mrs. McIntosh's involvement brings the students and their choral director many benefits, and the opportunity to work with them adds structure to her week. She schedules her activities around her accompaniment responsibilities, and she practices the music outside the rehearsals to ensure perfection. She enjoys her musical involvement with the students and the choral director, and the success she experiences with them contributes to the quality of her life. Mrs. McIntosh's work provides her a unique place in the community where she taught school for so many years, and she finds it particularly rewarding. She derives much satisfaction from her activities as she makes music a special part of the students' school experiences. The intergenerational relationships among Mrs. McIntosh, the choral director, and the students are mutually beneficial.

Intergenerational Music Programming in the Community

Additional intergenerational experiences come from community orchestras or bands, civic choirs, and other music activities. It is not unusual for people who play in a community band to range in age from 16 to 80. The older musicians serve as mentors to the younger ones, and all experience community traditions together for the community's benefit. One research study demonstrated the positive effects of intergenerational music with an examination of the attitudes of teenagers and older adults (Darrow, Johnson, & Ollenberger, 1994). The study group, comprising 27 high school students and 24 older people, sang in a school choir for the entire school year. In addition, they participated in choir-related activities. The results showed that the teenagers' attitudes about the older members of the choir improved over the year, as did the attitudes of the older adults regarding the teenagers. At the same time, the older adults' attitudes about themselves improved, especially for the men. This study indicates the potential for successful outcomes when musical ensembles are developed. In 1998, Bowers implemented a comparative study that examined the attitudes of college students and older adults in an intergenerational choral setting. Based on pretest and posttest scores from both the college students and the older adults, results from the study indicated that both age groups reported an increase in attitude towards the other age group.

Intergenerational Music Programming in the Residential Care Facility

Another community context for intergenerational programs is within residential care facilities for older adults. The residents of these facilities can range in age from 60 to over 100. Often, a range of 30–40 years exists among the residents' ages. Consequently, the residents are an intergenerational group. Along with the wide span of ages represented in residential care facilities comes the broad, varied experiences of the residents, and with these backgrounds comes the potential for making significant and interesting contributions to participation in music. It is essential to recognize the diversity among the residents and not to assume they are alike in their preference for music or participation in it. Each resident's age must be acknowledged and his or her musical preferences considered. Enlisting diversity can enhance musical experiences.

Considering the diversity among the residents of residential care facilities not only contributes to their quality of life but has significance for entire communities that have the wisdom to understand their value as preservers of traditions. Although some residents are physically frail, many of them are alert and cognitively functional. Communities can benefit only when these individuals are integrated into activities.

If the residents are too physically frail to leave the facility, then the community can go to them. Meetings of various clubs and organizations can be held at the care facilities so that residents who are members can attend with ease. Other community activities, including recitals, ensemble performances, and even rehearsals, can be integrated into the nursing facility. These activities can provide stimulation and continued engagement for all members of the community.

Many facets of community life and history can be shared as members of the community integrate with residents of residential care facilities. Individuals may describe music activities and traditions and may even perform some of the music with support and encouragement. The following example illustrates the sometimes surprising responses that are received from requests to share music from the past:

> Mrs. Janek, a nursing facility resident with late-stage dementia, was participating in a music therapy group session that included group singing. After one of the songs was completed, she suddenly stood up and began to sing in Russian a song she had sung all her life. Her daughter, who was also a participant at the session, held her mother's hand and sang with her. After the session, the daughter, who was in her 60s, was tearful as she said, "I have not heard Mother sing in years, and it was wonderful to have the opportunity to share that part of her life with her again."

Some residents have complete memories of music activities practiced in the community, and, if asked, they can provide oral histories of the community's music development and traditions. Often these oral histories include information specifically about people for whom there may be no other source of information. This was the case concerning a family in which all of the older members had died. A visit with a man in a residential care facility revealed some of the family's musical history:

> The conversation began with a question about an old pump organ that had been found in the attic of the family's farmhouse some years before and had been subsequently restored. The man said that he remembered the organ, and that it had been transported in a horse-drawn wagon to various homes in the community for musical events. It had a removable top, handles on the sides of the bottom portion, two manuals, pull stops, and two foot pedal pumps. The removable top, which was decorative and had no musical function, had not been transported. The men would carefully lift the bottom of the organ from the wagon by its handles and move it into the parlor for an evening of singing as a crowd of neighbors gathered.
>
> He described the music activities in which the organ was a vital part by saying, "There is an old story that I heard many times as a young boy about how that organ came to this community. Grandmother had just married, and Grandfather had the organ shipped by wagon all the way from St. Louis as her wedding present. When it arrived, Grandmother was so delighted that she pumped the pedals and played until she was exhausted! Word spread throughout the county, and people came from miles around to see this magnificent instrument.
>
> "You know, Grandmother was quite a fine player, and Uncle Pat played fiddle like nobody's business. The times with music on that organ at Grandmother's old farm homestead were the very best. Everyone would bring covered dishes. There would be fruit pies served with fresh cream so thick you could cut it with a knife, and fried chicken, mashed potatoes and gravy, and the best biscuits you ever ate. Of course, they were

tastiest with homemade butter piled on them and topped off with plum jam.

"People would come from all around, and as the women laid out the food, the men unhitched the horses. They watered and fed them as they settled them into the barn for the night. When the animals were cared for, the folks would gather around the big dining room table and fill their plates with food. There were so many people that they sat all around the house to eat. As soon as everyone was finished, the music would begin. Grandmother would begin to play that organ, Uncle Pat would fiddle along, and everyone would stomp their feet and clap. In just a little bit, they would all begin to dance, and it would seem as if the entire room was moving. I can remember feeling like the whole house was jumping up and down.

"These dancing parties would go on into the wee hours, and just when no one could go another set, Grandmother would pull the cover over the organ keys and retrieve the feather beds. Everyone would get the quilts and pillows they had brought from the wagons, and people would bed down all over the house for the night. Several adults would lay across each bed, the women in some rooms and the men in others. They made pallets on the floor for the children beside their mothers, and the young men all slept in the attic. The fun we used to have! Grandmother sure knew how to make a party!"

This man's description of the country parties put the living members of his family in touch with their roots in the community. The history seemed to come alive as he spoke. Whenever the pump organ is played, it is as if some of the people from the man's past are present, and that the old farmhouse could still pulsate with their dancing.

Residents of care facilities also may participate in music as audience members. There are perhaps no more accepting or tolerant audiences for musical performances than residents of care facilities. They accept efforts to perform or to make music graciously. This does not mean that they cannot or do not discriminate quality in performance. They have simply developed the wisdom to accept people at face value. Their nonjudgmental, supportive acceptance is particularly important for performers who may be somewhat timid or shy and need experience to build their confidence and to desensitize them to performance anxiety. These older audiences can be used to preview musical performances before they are given elsewhere. Junior high and high school students can perform solo and ensemble pieces before competitions, college and university students can perform their repertoires before recitals, jazz and popular music groups can play before they audition for paying jobs, and people who want to play an instrument or sing without stress and pressure from critics can enjoy performing before an audience of older adults. These performances also stimulate the audience intellectually and provide opportunities for social interactions. Through music, the performers and audience share benefits, and as music functions to enhance their lives, it contributes to the overall quality of their community.

PARTICIPATION IN MUSIC TO MAINTAIN TRADITIONS

Older people use music in a variety of ways in order to maintain traditions. These traditions may be certain music-training approaches, the traditions of particular cultures and ethnic groups, the traditions of making and repairing fine instruments, or the traditions that are preserved in music in family celebrations and other significant family events, as in the following example:

> Mr. Hennesey used music to celebrate his 85th birthday with his family. He had composed a song that included the significant events in his life, from his upbringing through his first job, his marriage to his wife of 64 years, and the births of his children, grandchildren, and great-grandchildren. He shared his feelings and thoughts about these events through his song. Mr. Hennesey recorded his music and made copies, which he presented to the members of his family after his performance. One of his daughters said later that she cherished her father's gift of song as one of the loveliest things he had ever given her.

Other traditions are maintained and passed on by music

teachers who studied with the masters and have firsthand experience of listening to and learning from great musicians. Whether these people are eminent classical, ethnic, or folk musicians, their legacy is lost without people who can pass on their approaches to making music. These living representatives may themselves be legendary in their talent and skills, and they nurture students and preserve music through their live performances, recordings, and teachings. These musicians may continue making musical contributions as they age, and thus serve as resources to the music community. This potential as a resource was demonstrated by a graduate of Julliard, who had taught music her entire adult life:

> Miss T., 96, died just after finishing a student's lesson. A friend found her sitting in a chair in her studio with a book on her lap and a serene expression on her face. She concluded her career quite peacefully, leaving behind the hundreds of musicians she had taught. People continue to hear her music because generations of her former students continue to perform it.

The legacy of Miss T. is not unusual. Many music teachers have contributed years of musical expression and enjoyment to their students and their students after them. Through music, they live on in many lives.

Another musical legacy is the art and skill of making and repairing the fine instruments used in performing. To create and maintain these valuable, even priceless, instruments requires the expertise of experienced craftspeople who are well trained in and have refined the techniques of instrument building and care. As these skilled technicians age, they become valued teachers who can train others in the traditions of musical instrument construction and maintenance. Not available in books, this training can come only from artisans who are willing to pass on their knowledge and skill to their successors. When these skilled craftspeople can no longer do the physical work themselves, they can describe or demonstrate the process in detail as they supervise others. The existence of fine instruments is preserved through these people, which makes a significant contribution to all communities.

PEER SUPPORT, OR "THE BUDDY SYSTEM"

Although some people may lack the courage to try something new alone, such as learning to sing, play, or read music, they may become more daring when they attempt to learn with a companion. A person may begin to study music with a friend who has also wanted to take music lessons. These people may not study the same instrument or even have the same teacher, but they can share the joys and frustrations of their new venture. One may encourage the other when progress seems slow, and one person can motivate the other by observing the advances made (i.e., people can be convinced of their own potential to develop musically when they observe others' successes).

Having a music "buddy" not only serves to motivate and encourage but can provide a partner for whom to perform or with whom to make music. Many hours can be delightfully filled with playing and/ or singing alone to develop skills and then together to share them, as in the following example:

> A woman who began studying piano in her 60s after giving up lessons as a child told a friend about her new interest. The woman's friend thought that studying music again after many years was a good idea, and she indicated that she would like to try the violin once more. The two friends began to learn and practice in earnest. After several months, they began to play simple duets and found their musical successes so stimulating that they encouraged other older adult friends to learn music. For these two people, mutual support led to hours of enjoyment. (Adams, 1995, p. 62)

If studying music or developing a musical skill is not of interest, numerous opportunities are available to actively participate with others in enjoying music. People may gather to listen to music either at home or at community musical events. Interests in particular types of music can be pursued at the local public library, and civic groups or organizations can be encouraged to schedule musical programs that can be shared by the entire community. Individuals may decide to sponsor the development of musical interests in the community and may organize concerts, recitals, and lectures for other interested people.

CONCLUSION

At some level of participation, music is available and accessible to most individuals who have an interest in it. Some people have the desire to learn or relearn musical skills, whereas others are content to be listeners. Whatever the desire, individuals must not allow age to preclude opportunities. The potential for satisfying musical experiences is great, and the active pursuit of many, varied experiences is encouraged.

REFERENCES

Adams, J. (1995). Strike up the music—and the memories. Piano lessons are far more rewarding now than they were during the author's childhood. *New Choices for Retirement Living*, 35(5), 60–63.

Bernard, A. (1992). The use of music as a purposeful activity: A preliminary investigation. *Physical and Occupational Therapy in Geriatrics*, 26(5), 99–141.

Bolton, C. (1985). Lifestyle management, proaction, and educational efficacy. *Educational Gerontology*, 11(4&5), 181–190.

Bowers, J. (1998). Effects of intergenerational choir for community-based senior and college students on age-related attitudes. *Journal of Music Therapy*, 35(1), 2–18.

Bowles, C. L. (1991). Self-expressed adult music education interests and music experiences. *Journal of Research in Music Education*, 39(3), 191–205.

Bruhn, H. (2002, Spring). Music development of elderly people. *Psychomusicology—A Journal of Research in Music Cognition*, 18, 59–75.

Coffman, D. (2002, Fall). Music and quality of life in older adults. *Psychomusicology—A Journal of Research in Music Cognition*, 18, 76–88.

Darrow, A. A., Johnson, C., & Ollenberger, T. (1994). The effect of participation in an intergenerational choir on teens' and older persons' cross-age attitudes. *Journal of Music Therapy*, 31(2), 119–134.

Feldman, P. H., & Oberlink, M. R. (2003). Developing community indicators to promote the health and well-being of older people. *Family & Community Health*, 26(2), 268–274.

Gibbons, A. C. (1982a). Musical Aptitude Profile scores in a non-institutionalized elderly population. *Journal of Research in Music Education*, 30(1), 23–29.

Gibbons, A. C. (1982b). A musical skill level self-evaluation in non-institutionalized elderly. *Activities, Adaptation & Aging*, 3(1), 61–67.

Gibbons, A. C. (1983). Primary Measures of Music Audiation scores in an institutionalized elderly population. *Journal of Music Therapy*, 20(1), 21–29.

Gibbons, A. C. (1984). A program for non-institutionalized mature adults: A description. *Activities, Adaptation & Aging*, 6(1), 71–80.

Greenfield, E. A., & Marks, N. F. (2007). Continuous participation in voluntary groups as a protective factor for the psychological well-being of adults who develop functional limitations: Evidence from the national survey of families and households. *The Journals of Gerontology*, 62B(1), S60–68.

Jellison, J. A. (1999). Life beyond the jingle stick: Real music in a real world. *Update: Applications of Research in Music Education*, 17(2), 13–19.

Johnson, G., Otto, D., & Clair, A. A. (2001). The effect of instrumental and vocal music on adherence to a physical rehabilitation exercise program with persons who are elderly. *Journal of Music Therapy*, 38(2), 82–96.

Koga, M. (2005). The music making and wellness project. *The American Music Teacher*, 55(2), 40–41.

Mathews, R. M., Clair, A. A., & Kosloski, K. (2001). Keeping the beat: Use of rhythmic music during exercise activities for the elderly with dementia. *American Journal of Alzheimer's Disease*, 16(6), 377–380.

Moore, R., Staum, M., & Brotons, M. (1992). Music preferences of the elderly: Repertoire, vocal ranges, tempos, and accompaniments for singing. *Journal of Music Therapy*, 29(4), 236–252.

Okun, M., Olding, R., & Cohn, C. (1990). A meta-analysis of subjective well-being interventions among elders. *Psychological Bulletin*, 108(2), 257–266.

VanWeelden, K., & Whipple, J. (2004). Effect of field experiences on music therapy students' perceptions of choral music for geriatric wellness programs. *Journal of Music Therapy*, 41(2), 340–352.

World Health Organization. (2001). *International classification of functioning, disability and health*. Geneva, Switzerland: Author.

Chapter 3

Therapeutic Music with People who have Dementia

Therapeutic Music with People who have Dementia

Dementia is often progressive in older people; it is certainly progressive if it is Alzheimer's-type dementia, a disease first described by Alois Alzheimer in 1907 (Whitehouse, 1992). A diagnosis of dementia must not be made without a thorough medical examination and evaluation by a geriatrician who has training and knowledge regarding dementias and their effects. Without rigorous medical testing, individuals with reactions to medications, infections, or other health problems may be misdiagnosed. If dementia is diagnosed, it is essential to know its cause and course so that appropriate interventions can be implemented and long-term care can be planned. In addition, it is essential for spouses and families to seek immediate legal counsel regarding health, property, and financial management.

The level of dementia is defined by functional abilities. Reisberg, Ferris, and Franssen (1985) have defined primary degenerative dementia as having stages, from mild forgetfulness to the inability to ambulate, eat, or speak. They define progressive dementia as the gradual loss of physical, emotional, and social abilities. When dysfunction progresses to the point that people can no longer have their health care and personal safety needs met at home, placement in residential care is inevitable.

It is estimated that in 2000 the number of individuals living with Alzheimer's in the United States was 4.5 million (Hebert, Scherr, Bienias, Bennett, & Evans, 2003). Dementia is the most common factor in the placement of older adults in nursing facilities (Hendrie, 1998). The incidence of this disease and other dementias is increasing because people are living longer and manifesting these illnesses later in life. Estimates indicate that each year even more people will be diagnosed with dementia as the population continues to age (Edland, Rocca, Petersen, Cha, & Kokmen, 2002). Studies indicate that without advances in therapy, the number of individuals with Alzheimer's is projected to rise to 13.2 million by the year 2050 (Hebert et al., 2003).

EARLY-STAGE DEMENTIA

Indications

The onset of dementia is often so subtle that it is not distinguishable until the disease has progressed and caregivers and family members think back over the past several years. It begins with a loss of memory for little things that are common in most people, with or without dementia. The difference lies in the progression to increased forgetfulness, disorientation, and confusion ("Dementia," 2003; Finkel, Costa, Silva, Cohen, Miller, & Sartorius, 1996).

Caregivers may remark about changes they see in the older person that they do not understand. Spouses may describe changes in disposition, often marked by gruffness, abruptness, and angry speech. These changes are particularly alarming to spouses who have had satisfying, loving relationships in which none of these aberrant behaviors was displayed. Adult children may describe a parent who was always efficient and fastidious, but who gradually became forgetful and disheveled, as in the following vignette:

> When I used to go see my mother, she was always so cheerful. The house was neat as a pin, and she seemed so glad to see me. I began to notice that she was getting forgetful, but I didn't think anything about it. Forgetfulness just happens to lots of people eventually, but something else has happened to Mom. She has become gradually worse. She doesn't seem to remember things that have just happened. Recently, I went to visit and there was a new, very expensive vacuum sweeper in the middle of the living room. When I asked about it, she said that she didn't remember exactly how she got it, but that some nice young man came to visit. When I checked her bank statement with her check registry, I found she had written a sizable check to a door-to-door salesman. In addition, she had made several large purchases at stores around town for things she would never use. She bought satin sheets for a waterbed, and she doesn't even have one, for heaven's sake! I also found she had been giving money away to charities all over town in checks of $100. All of this is very strange since Mom has always been so thrifty. But it's not only the money. She has just let herself go. Last time I dropped in for a visit I found her with no makeup on, her hair in a mess, and food stains down the front of her dress. She looked horrible, and that's just not like Mom. She always did her hair and her makeup, even if

she was going to do housework all day. I also found partially eaten food around the house, even in her bedroom. When I asked what was going on with her, she just smiled and said, "Whatever do you mean? Everything is fine, dear. Don't you worry about a thing." I know something is terribly wrong with my mother. She has become so erratic and irresponsible that I am afraid to leave her alone.

Caregivers also may report decisions made regarding financial matters that are opposed to the values their loved ones have always held. They may find withdrawals of large amounts of money from savings or investment accounts, substantial loans for business ventures, sudden retirement without explanation, or other activities that may have serious or harmful consequences.

In addition to erratic behavior, symptoms of depression are often precursors to a diagnosis of dementia (Gatz, Tyas, St. John, & Montgomery, 2005). These symptoms may be the first indication to caregivers that a serious condition exists. At this point, caregivers usually insist that their loved ones receive medical examinations to determine the cause of the depression. A diagnosis of dementia may result.

Once diagnosed, people with dementia generally understand enough to know what is happening to them, and they may even know the expected course of their disease. They find themselves in a situation far beyond their control, helpless, and with no recourse. Thus, depression is almost inevitable. Depression presents serious health concerns and requires intervention (Iliffe, Manthorpe, & Eden, 2003; Kales, Blow, Copeland, Bingham, Kammerer, & Mellow, 1999). These concerns stem from a person's lack of appetite and subsequent poor nutrition; sleep disruptions; resistance to performing activities of daily living (ADLs), such as taking medications and bathing; lack of participation in activities that were once meaningful and contributed to quality of life, especially if these activities require complex processing; general apathy; and even threats of suicide. Medical attention and pharmacological management of the symptoms are necessary to ensure individual safety and well-being. Other interventions, such as music therapy, which provide opportunities for successful experiences and feelings of accomplishment, can also enhance quality of life during depressive episodes.

When symptoms of depression lift, people with dementia may engage in obsessive activities, such as looking about the house for an object they have misplaced, emptying drawers or shelves, or moving continually. These activities may provide them with some sense of control over their environment and may provide structure because they are performing simple, familiar tasks. These behaviors may also provide a way to do something purposeful, which may be particularly important to people who have a history of active engagement in work or involvement in home improvement projects. These individuals probably understand that they are progressively losing their capacity to function independently, and their behavior may be a way to maintain some sense of usefulness and integrity as a viable member of the household. Thus, these repetitive, obsessive behaviors have a calming effect on people with dementia, but they can irritate caregivers. Any attempts by caregivers to end the behaviors may precipitate disturbed reactions. Thus, often, caregivers sacrifice their own comfort and tolerate the chaotic household in order to promote calm and tranquility.

Interventions

Spouses and family members may or may not seek intervention as a loved one begins to display symptoms of early-stage dementia. Their openness to intervention depends greatly upon their willingness to accept the disease diagnosis and its prognosis. Often, spouses and other family members initially deny the inevitable course of the disease, but eventually they recognize that their loved one's behavior is changing. Some caregivers may decide to care for their loved ones at home. In general, they make every effort to carry out ADLs much as they did before the disease symptoms appeared.

Once depression and other symptoms of dementia become evident, the most common intervention is pharmacological management. Although there is no cure for dementia, physicians can prescribe medications that may have some effect on reducing the symptoms (Ringman & Cummings, 2006). Physicians may also recommend involvement in support groups for both caregivers and care recipients. The groups act as a network of people who can provide information and encouragement throughout the disease process. Group members can help caregivers and care recipients cope with and resolve the grief associated with the onset of dementia. Group members are also insiders, people who have first-hand experience with the disease. This experience makes them able to empathize completely, no matter what the circumstance. Contact with these people provides the hope and consolation that is necessary for survival (Snyder, Jenkins, & Joosten, 2007; Zarit, Femia, Watson, Rice-Oeschger, & Kakos, 2004).

Because of the prominence of depression in early-stage dementia, it may not be possible to encourage people with the disease to actively produce music. However, music can be used in other ways to enhance the quality of life of older people. Hanser (1990) used music therapy interventions to relieve depression in older adults. Her approach included using music therapy techniques in exercise, relaxation, facial massage, positive imagery, and creative expression. After an initial assessment of each individual's needs, Hanser tailored a music therapy program to meet those needs. Each participant was asked to use the program at home daily for a period of 8 weeks. Hanser also visited each person once a week during the 8 weeks to assist in implementing the program. At the end of the 8-week trial, Hanser found significant changes in the symptoms of depression. She concluded that the music therapy program could be successfully employed at home after training was provided by a music therapist.

Early in the disease process, the use of music may relieve fear and some symptoms of depression by structuring time and providing an opportunity for some meaningful participation in activities in which people with dementia may still successfully engage (Ashida, 2000). Participation is most effective when it uses skills that have been practiced over many years, have personal significance, and are still accessible. For example, prompting people who have regularly played an instrument to play a favorite song on the instrument may lift their spirits and occupy them. Also, singing with people who have always enjoyed singing may divert their attention and contribute to a positive shift in mood, as in the following vignette:

> Mrs. Graves seemed to become depressed when she was not occupied around the house. Whenever her husband noticed her quietness and sad face, he sat beside her, took her hand,

and sang "their song." Usually within a phrase or two she joined him. Her eyes brightened, her brow smoothed, and she smiled. His song therapy successfully distracted her from a gloomy moment.

People with early-stage dementia also can participate successfully in group music activities, which may include singing in a church choir or a community chorale, or dancing (Palo-Bengtsson, Winblad, & Ekman, 1998). Ballroom and square dancing are particularly successful forms of dance because both have simple, repetitive steps. Attendance at community dances sponsored by the parks and recreation department; senior centers; or organizations such as the Fraternal Order of Eagles, the Moose Lodge, Veterans of Foreign Wars, or the American Legion can be enjoyable and beneficial. Even dancing at home while the radio plays may be satisfying to a person with dementia and his or her partner.

Whether music is used individually or in groups of people it, provides some opportunities for people with dementia to compensate for their disabilities. People perform much as they always have, provided the performance is contingent upon skills that do not require complex cognitive processing. These skills remain in the behavioral repertoire for a long time (Beatty et al., 1988). Access to these skills likely occurs automatically, through years of usage, and is triggered by the familiarity of the music (Cuddy & Duffin, 2005). The structure and order inherent in the music support participating in it and allow individuals to function with purpose and meaning. However, as their disease progresses, they will require support to continue participating in music, as follows:

Mr. Hawkins played the trumpet in jazz ensembles all his adult life. Because of his dementia, he could no longer drive to the job venues. One of the band members offered to drive him. Although Mr. Hawkins could not remember the names of the musicians in the band, once he was on the bandstand, he played with fine quality and accuracy. Occasionally he switched to another tune, apparently miscued by a note sequence or other musical component. With musical cues provided by the pianist, he generally switched back to the original tune without apparent distress. The support provided by his fellow musicians allowed Mr. Hawkins to extend his career as a professional musician.

Using music is not intended as a method to avoid discussing the feelings associated with coping with dementia, but as an occasional respite from coping with the disease process. In addition, the satisfaction derived from successful participation in a familiar activity promotes feelings of well-being. Successful participation in music demonstrates competencies, relieves frustrations, calms, brightens mood, and diminishes feelings of failure for a time (Sixsmith & Gibson, 2006).

As people move into later stages of dementia, the skills that require cognitive memory, discrimination, and integration are progressively eliminated. For example, people who have a history of playing the guitar or piano begin to forget how to finger chords and may give up playing, greatly frustrated and indignant. Other people may not be able to read notation for a new piece of music but are able to play along when familiar tunes are played. Others may discreetly give up their instrumental performances but still participate in music by singing, dancing, or playing a drum. These skills will also be lost as people progress through the stages of the disease, but the uses of music can be altered to suit changing levels of physical, psychological, and social response. Consequently, musical experiences can be successful and apparently pleasing to individuals through the later stages of dementia.

MIDDLE-STAGE DEMENTIA

Indications

Reisberg et al. (1985) have defined people in middle-stage dementia as needing help with ADLs; being unable to remember a spouse's name; being unaware of recent events; displaying anxious, agitated, delusional, or obsessive behavior; having disturbed sleep patterns (staying awake at night and sleeping during the day); experiencing emotional changes; being unable to carry on conversations; and being unable to follow through with tasks.

People with middle-stage dementia may eventually create severe management problems in the home. In their confusion, people with dementia may become physically combative and aggressive because they may think that their caregiver is a stranger who is trying to harm them. They may beg to go home, even though they are in the home in which they have lived for many years. They may refuse all efforts to bathe, feed, or adequately clothe them, and they may be physically and verbally abusive. In many ways, they pose a serious threat to their own safety and the safety of their caregivers. When people with dementia become so much of a burden that the caregiver becomes physically ill, emotionally drained, or otherwise unable to cope, it becomes necessary to place them in a residential facility equipped with adequate staff and the physical resources necessary to provide for them (Knopman, Berg, Thomas, Grundman, Thal, & Sano,1999; Smith, Kokmen, & O'Brien, 2000).

Other individuals with middle-stage dementia may no longer possess the facility with language to ask comprehensible questions or to successfully communicate verbally at all. They may use "word salad" (disjointed word or sentence fragments), which makes it difficult to interact with them (Savundranayagam, Hummert, & Montgomery, 2005). When they are misunderstood, they can become frustrated and have outbursts of anger.

People with middle-stage dementia also have extremely short attention spans that disrupt everything they attempt to do. Attention deficits increase as social and cognitive functions decline. Eventually, these people need assistance with ADLs.

Interventions

Quality of Life Programs

When people with dementia require residential placement, these facilities must provide quality of life programs that go beyond meeting physical needs for care and safety. These institutions are mandated by the federal government to "promote care for residents in a manner and in an environment that maintains or enhances each resident's dignity and respect in full recognition of his or her individuality" (Rules and Regulations 48871, 1991). In addition, the federal Omnibus Budget Reconciliation Act of 1987, also commonly known as the Nursing Home Reform Act, mandates activities that meet the interests and the needs for physical, mental, and psychosocial well-being of each resident (Omnibus Budget Reconciliation Act, 1987). These facilities must provide quality of life programs in order to remain certified by the Health Care Financing Administration for Medicare and Medicaid reimbursements.

All residential care facilities must meet licensure requirements in their respective states in order to provide care that is funded by Medicare and Medicaid. In each state, these requirements must comply with the federal mandates to promote care that maintains or enhances dignity while respecting and recognizing each resident's individuality. To meet these requirements, facilities must provide ongoing activity programs for residents. However, efforts to provide these programs are generally met with frustration by individuals who have attempted to involve people with cognitive, social, and physical dysfunction in purposeful, meaningful activities. To avoid such frustration, musical experiences can be designed to meet a wide range of response levels and can enhance the functioning abilities that remain in people with dementia.

These abilities may not be apparent at the time of placement because of relocation stress (Anderson, Beaver, & Culliton, 1996). Relocation stress occurs when a change in residence results in added agitation or other problem behaviors (Aneshenel, Pearlin, Levy-Storms, & Schuler, 2000). The frustration felt by new residents in trying to remember how to find the restroom or how to recognize their own bed may be translated into behaviors that range from withdrawal to open confrontation. Often a structured environment with a regimented daily schedule can make some people feel more comfortable. In addition, permission to wander unrestricted through certain protected areas in the facility seems to relieve some agitation. Attempts to integrate individuals into activities that family members have indicated are favorites sometimes engage attention and purposeful participation. Frequent attention from the same staff members seems to reassure and encourage active interaction with others.

Even if people with dementia seem to recognize caregivers by their faces or usual clothing, they may have progressed far enough in the disease that they do not always recognize their spouses, or if they do recognize them, they may not call them by name. They may not recognize other members of their immediate family at all. They may not be able to discriminate delusion from reality and may have hallucinations. People with dementia tend to walk with their heads and eyes down and do not acknowledge other people in proximity to them. Often, they bump into other residents or staff, which may result in physical combativeness and aggression. Their postures may be altered by damage to the motor areas of the brain, which results in leaning forward or backward while walking, shuffling gait, lowering one shoulder, difficulty in locomotion, and pain and discomfort. Often, people with dementia are cold because of brain damage that causes inadequate body temperature regulation (Lucero, 1995).

Often, people with middle-stage dementia are totally disoriented to time and place, and usually they do not remember even significant events in their lives. They may ask when people who are long deceased are coming to visit. They may want to know where their mother has gone. They may claim that another resident is their child and attempt to feed or bathe the resident. Some individuals may ask what day it is, what time it is, or where they are. Providing the information is usually reassuring, but they may ask the same question repeatedly because they cannot remember that they asked or that they received an answer. The appropriate approach with these people is to look directly at them, make eye contact if they can tolerate it, and clearly and calmly provide the requested information.

Attempts at reality orientation in some people in middle-stage dementia are denied, ignored, or reacted to with anger or more harmful emotions. With memory loss, information concerning past events is new each time it is heard, and the grief associated with it is as intense as it was the first time it was experienced. The appropriate approach with these people is to meet their needs in ways that are most conducive to their comfort levels. Naomi Feil's validation therapy (Feil, 1993) is often the most efficacious. Her approach involves treating people with dementia with an attitude of respect while providing them with an empathic listener who does not judge but accepts their view of reality. The following is a good example of how effective validation can be:

> Mr. Tierney approached the nurses' station at the nursing facility in which he lived and asked when his wife was coming to

take him home. Tisha, a nursing assistant, replied that his wife could not be there right now, that she was delayed by some things she had to do at home. Tisha then asked Mr. Tierney if he would like some company for a while. He indicated that he would, and she put her arm around his shoulder, walked him over to the couch, and sat down beside him for a few minutes. She asked Mr. Tierney if he would like something to drink. He remained calm as she left him for a moment to get a glass of juice. When she returned, she talked with him about his day and encouraged him to participate in the activity in the day room. He willingly went with her to the activity group. The other residents immediately captured Mr. Tierney's attention, and he joined them. Tisha returned to her duties at the nurses' station.

This approach allowed Tisha to address Mr. Tierney's need to assuage his loneliness while distracting him. His wife had died some years before, but he did not remember. For Tisha to tell him that his wife would not be coming to get him, that in fact she is dead, would likely result in either vehement denial or crying, agitation, and perhaps physical combativeness so extreme that tranquilizers may be required to calm him.

Though validation may seem appropriate with certain individuals, it is always important to obtain family approval before using it. Some family members are strongly opposed to the validation approach on the basis that it is not truthful. These family members insist that their loved ones be told truthful facts in all cases, no matter their reactions.

Music Therapy

People with middle-stage dementia can still participate in music (Cevasco & Grant, 2006; Takahashi & Matsushita, 2006). Music provides structured reality, order, and predictability. It brings something familiar to the environment, and individuals indicate their recognition of it through pleasant facial expressions and vocal responses. Music gives meaning to their environment when so many other experiences are not understandable (Whitcomb, 1989). People with dementia may respond spontaneously to music by tapping their feet, clapping, or dancing. Some research has demonstrated that people can participate in structured music therapy sessions for as long as 30 minutes (Clair & Bernstein, 1990a), and that they participate in music longer than they do in another commonly used activity, listening to someone reading to them (Clair, 1996; Groene, 1993). They can participate for a long period of time—15 months or more—even when their cognitive, social, and physiological abilities continue to deteriorate. In these music therapy sessions, people may watch others play rhythm instruments, participate themselves either spontaneously or with cues, and interact successfully with others in a socially acceptable form (Clair & Bernstein, 1990b). People with dementia may use music as an iconic representation of the feelings they can no longer express in words (Aldridge, 1995). For example, they may beat loudly and furiously on drums or strum a guitar softly as it is laid across their lap. Music offers ways to access and maintain cognitive and affective functioning, even when people are severely impaired (Lipe, 1991), as well as ways to socially interact with others (Clair & Bernstein, 1990b; Lynch, 1987). Social interaction during music therapy may even encourage social contact after the session (Pollack & Namazi, 1992). Music can be a viable addition to many activities in which attention focus and cooperative behaviors are desired.

In general, music from the past that is familiar and is associated with positive experiences and memories is the most likely to evoke responses. As dementia progresses, the music that evokes responses changes from that which was popular in the adult years to that which was popular in early childhood. Initially, music preferred throughout adulthood will facilitate commitment to and engagement in participation in music. People with dementia who liked and listened to popular music and were active consumers of it generally prefer the popular music of their young adult years to the popular music of later periods of adult life (Gibbons, 1977; Groene, 2001). This music was the music that they listened to while courting, attending dances, and sitting at home or at the soda fountain. Some people may even have played an instrument or sung in a band.

Other people with dementia may have been avid listeners of classical music and opera. They may have attended concerts and other performances regularly throughout their lifetime. Although some of these people were also listeners of popular music, a number of them may never have developed a taste for it. Thus, popular music would not likely produce desirable responses in these individuals.

Whatever music is preferred will be the most effective in promoting interest in and commitment to participation, as long as the memory of the music remains intact. When the brain can no longer retrieve experiences associated with preferred music throughout adulthood, it can still generally access music learned earlier in life, including traditional folk songs learned in school and ethnic music that was part of family life. This music carries with it a full range of well-integrated associations, emotions, and memories. Satisfying experiences with it are immediate and do not require cognitive processing for success. Suggestions for these applications are provided by several authors, including Bright (1988), Chavin (1991), Douglass (1985), Shaw (1993), and Aldridge (2000). Program information that includes planning and implementing music therapy for people with dementia is provided by Gfeller and Hanson (1995).

Singing. People with severe cognitive impairment may not participate in singing if the range of notes is too high (Moore, Staum, & Brotons, 1992) or if the tempos are so fast that they do not allow time to articulate the words (Douglass, 1985; Moore et al., 1992). Often, sheet music is pitched too high for older people to sing comfortably. Moore and colleagues (1992) suggest transposing songs into lower keys—between F3 and C5 for women and nearly an octave lower for men. Tempos must be slowed from those generally used to make singing easier (Clair & Bernstein, 1989). These recommendations indicate a need for spontaneity that is available only with live accompaniments, which can be adjusted in pitch, tempo, and volume in order to facilitate singing experiences. One of the best instruments for such accompaniments is the acoustic guitar (Bright, 1981; Douglass, 1985; Moore et al., 1992), and the accompanist must have sufficient skill with the instrument to adjust playing as needed.

Even with making adjustments to vocal ranges and tempos, observation shows that as dementia progresses, people can no longer sing the lyrics of the songs they knew as young adults. They may react to familiar songs (Brotons, 2000; Olderog Millard & Smith, 1989; Sung & Chang, 2005) and can sing the melodies of familiar songs, but the words are forgotten (Christie, 1992). The lyrics may not have been practiced often enough to be integrated into their musical memories. For a time, sheet music may facilitate participation in singing, but eventually people with dementia lose the ability to read. When this occurs, sheet music becomes a distraction or even a source of frustration and preoccupation that impedes participation. Singing songs that were learned early in life is still possible (Bright, 1992; Clair & Bernstein, 1989; Prickett & Moore, 1991; Ridder & Aldridge, 2005; Whitcomb, 1993). These songs include folk songs, patriotic songs, and hymns that were learned in school, at home, or in a religious setting. Because these songs were so well integrated into people's lives, they remain in the memory longer than songs learned later in life. Although many of these songs were learned in childhood, songs that appeal to young children, such as "Mary Had a Little Lamb" and "Old McDonald Had a Farm," may not be appropriate for older adults because they may harm self-esteem. However, songs such as "Row, Row, Row Your Boat" may be received with enthusiasm, and "Home on the Range," "Oh! Susanna," and "She'll Be Comin' 'Round the Mountain" may be even better at encouraging participation. The most effective songs of all may be songs sung in a person's native language or songs that were sung by a parent or grandparent.

It is a popular belief that people with degenerative dementia can continue to sing even when they can no longer speak. Although singing in some form continues for certain persons through late-stage dementia, research shows that many people discontinue singing sometime in the middle stage of the disease (Clair, 1991; Clair & Bernstein, 1990a). It is not possible to predict the exact time because it occurs at a different time for each individual in the degenerative process. Before singing ceases altogether, some individuals may vocalize while others sing. These sounds seem to be attempts to trace the contour of the melody for a given song, but accurate pitch matching and lyrics are not employed. For other individuals, their vocalizations do not resemble singing, except that they occur while others sing and apparently are not indications of distress or pain. These responses are purposeful, however, and should be encouraged as engagements in active participation.

Dancing. Even when singing and speaking have stopped with the progression of the dementia, individuals can still move rhythmically to music (Palo-Bengtsson et al., 1998). Often, people who danced as young adults respond to music that has a definite, accented beat, particularly if it is familiar, by moving their feet and/or swinging their arms in time to the music. If they do not make these movements spontaneously, they will participate readily if someone takes their hands or moves with them into a couple's ballroom dance position. They can hold a partner and move their feet in time to the music, even when their ability to ambulate has diminished and they have lost the ability to speak coherently or at all.

Dancing is a particularly effective way for caregiving spouses to once again experience emotional closeness with their loved ones (Palo-Bengtsson & Ekman, 2000). A research study of four couples in which one member of each couple had been diagnosed with probable Alzheimer's disease indicated that ballroom dancing was a viable and desirable way for couples to interact (Clair, Tebb, & Bernstein, 1993). These couples, who met as a group once a week for 8 weeks, danced well together, although the people with dementia were confused and generally unable to carry on conversations with their spouses. These couples had danced together earlier in their lives but had no recent dancing experiences until the music therapy program was implemented. The music therapy sessions provided the opportunity to again enjoy dancing, not only during the sessions but outside them as well. One woman excitedly approached the music therapists before one of the sessions and said:

> My husband came into the kitchen one afternoon this week while I was preparing lunch. The radio was playing a rather bouncy tune, and he held out his arms and asked, "Dance?" I immediately stopped what I was doing and went into his arms. I was so delighted that he wanted to dance with me, and that he initiated it! We've been dancing in the kitchen ever since! I don't think he would have tried the dancing if we hadn't done it here in the music therapy group.

The music therapy program of Clair et al. and subsequent observations of other couples like those in the study have demonstrated that dancing successfully engages spouses as a couple. Dancing in middle-stage dementia offers an opportunity for the well spouse to be held in the arms of his or her loved one. This emotionally intimate experience is generally missing in the relationship by the middle stage of the disease process. A wife who danced with her husband of 50 years during a music therapy session on a dementia care unit was found crying outside of the unit after the session. When approached by the music therapist, the wife said, "You have no idea what you have done. My husband has not held me for 3+ years, until today, and I have missed him so. Thank you for giving me that." This caregiver's response to the emotional closeness she sensed when she danced with her husband has been incorporated into other music therapy interventions for caregiving and care receiving spouses who participate as couples. The responses received indicate the spouses' great satisfaction at the opportunity to do something that has not been accessible to them for some time with their loved ones. Caregiving spouses also make remarks such as the following:

> I have been pleasantly surprised by my wife when music therapy is the purpose of my visit with her. She can still dance with me, and though she gets distracted from time to time, I can easily get her attention again. When we're dancing I feel like she is here with me. This is very different from our usual visits, when I spend most of my time just following her as she wanders around the special care unit. (Clair & Ebberts, 1997)

When dancing is not possible because of religious convictions or physical limitations, it is still possible to have close physical contact using music. Caregiving spouses, children, or other family members can sit beside their loved ones and hold hands, link arms, or put arms about the waist or shoulders. They may or may not lean their heads together and rock from side to side while the music plays. Entire families may sit in a circle holding hands or wrap their arms around one another and sway with the music. Others may sit face to face with legs to either side. They may wrap their arms about one another and sway to music cheek to cheek or with the head on the partner's chest. One adult daughter put her arms around her mother as they stood and swayed to the rhythm of the music (Clair & Ebberts, 1997). These and other methods of promoting physical closeness will help meet the needs of both caregivers and care recipients for emotional intimacy. However, any form of physical closeness must take into consideration comfort levels and past experiences of emotional expression for people with dementia and the people who love them. The need for privacy must be respected in order to encourage responsiveness, and either recorded music or music sung by the caregivers may establish a context for closeness.

For people with dementia who pull away when physical closeness is attempted and for people who have no experience with dancing, holding hands with another person often stimulates the swinging of arms in time to music. Sometimes these individuals rock from foot to foot when both their hands are grasped and they are cued through role modeling to do so. These rhythmic responses occur commonly because they do not require complex cognitive functioning in order to facilitate success.

Using Rhythm. Several researchers have shown that people with severe debilitation in middle-stage dementia can still participate in music with other people by using rhythm (Cevasco & Grant, 2006). This participation in rhythm includes entrainment (playing in synchrony with others) (Hart, 1990); playing freely alone or while others play; and imitating the rhythms of others (Groene, 2001), with progressive accuracy and complexity over time (Clair, Bernstein, & Johnson, 1995; Clair & Ebberts, 1997). Research also shows that this participation does not continue without structure and guidance, but occurs in response to the actions of a music therapist, who carefully programs the stimulus to elicit the responses (Clair et al., 1995). Other research shows that people tend to participate longer in applications that involve vibrotactile stimulation rather than in those that do not (Clair & Bernstein, 1990a; Clair & Bernstein, 1993), and longer when playing drums than when singing or moving to music (Ebberts, 1994). Consequently, playing drums that are in the lap or large drums that emit strong vibrations and loud sounds tends to promote longer periods of participation in music in people with severe dementia than do other music applications (Clair et al., 1995). These instruments have discrete sounds that clearly begin when the instruments are struck. This clarity makes possible definite discrimination of the rhythmic beat, a prerequisite to participation in rhythm.

The author's observations show that participation with rhythm is sometimes spontaneous and seems almost automatic. When individuals with severe dementia are handed a mallet, which they reach for with their dominant hand, and then a drum, which they hold in their nondominant hand, they often begin to play even without receiving a request to do so. However, they generally do not continue participating without the structure provided by a music therapist. If this structure is provided through visual models to imitate and verbal cues to play, they continue to drum. Often, they quickly adapt, or entrain, their individual beats to one another. These people, who can no longer carry on intelligible, verbal conversations; who have hallucinations and delusions; who tend to isolate from others; and who do not perform ADLs independently, can still interact purposefully using rhythm.

Research demonstrates that applications of rhythm provide a means of escaping isolation and interacting with others, even when the cognitive, social, and emotional abilities to do so are gone (Brotons & Pickett-Cooper, 1994). They likely provide this opportunity because little or no cognitive processing is required to feel or tap out a beat. Rhythm is the basis of most activity and the ability to feel or tap out a rhythm remains intact in people with dementia for a long time.

Although playing percussion instruments is engaging for some people, it is contraindicated for others. Some people may react with pain to loud noise and others may respond with increased agitation. However, the author has observed that most people appear to settle into a relaxed state while participating in structured, predictable patterns of playing. Other people may indicate that they are not interested in playing. These people must be allowed to exercise their right not to participate.

Using Music Implemented by Caregivers. Some music therapies designed and implemented by music therapists for people with dementia can be used by caregivers to relieve boredom, avoid agitation, and increase their loved one's opportunities for involvement in music (Clair, 2002; Gotell, Brown, & Ekman, 2000). Music therapists may consult with caregivers and their care recipients to design programs that incorporate caregivers' musical skills and to train caregivers to use the programs when the services of a music therapist are not available. These programs can incorporate singing, drumming, and dancing. The effectiveness of such a music therapy program has been demonstrated, and a caregiver training program has been developed (Clair & Ebberts, 1997).

Music therapists may record an audiotape tailored to the vocal range and tempo of a particular care recipient. The tape may include the music therapist singing, or it may simply provide musical accompaniment for singing. The tape may include the individual's favorite songs, which may or may not be introduced or cued verbally, depending on the individual's cognitive abilities to understand. Caregivers may use the tape during the periods of the day when care recipients become restless, agitated, or bored.

Music therapists may also make interactive videos for individuals with dementia. These videos can include songs, rhythm applications, and other simple music participation tasks tailored to individuals' skills and response levels. New videos can be made available as skills and abilities change over time. These videos are more successful in individuals who have participated in music therapy sessions in which the applications were used. The videos provide a follow-up to sessions using familiar tasks and music. The music therapist conducts a session designed for a particular person, asking the individual to perform various tasks and modeling the tasks as the instructions are given. The pace is that which is the most appropriate for the individual, and sufficient time for the care recipient to respond is incorporated. Verbal feedback is also provided by calling the individual by name.

LATE-STAGE DEMENTIA

Indications and Interventions

Late-stage dementia is characterized by a loss of verbal articulation and physical ambulation, along with bowel and bladder incontinence (Reisberg et al., 1985). People in this stage are withdrawn, may sleep for long periods of time, and may be unresponsive to most stimuli. Efforts to provide for quality of life are still important for people in late-stage dementia. Programming that contributes to their dignity is federally mandated (Rules and Regulations 48871, 1991;

Omnibus Budget Reconciliation Act, 1987). In general, these efforts involve caring for physical needs by feeding the residents, keeping them clean and dry, maintaining the integrity of their skin, and providing medical interventions for any illnesses.

Individuals with cognitive losses do not participate in regularly offered activities and require specialized interventions that may not be routinely offered (Voelkl, Fries, & Galecki, 1995). To provide some opportunities for activity, residential care staff often use tape-recorded background music or bedside radios. Although this music can provide needed stimulation, it can be harmful if it does not match the musical taste of the individual who must listen to it or if it plays incessantly. Information about a resident's musical preferences can be obtained from spouses or other family members. If these sources are not available or if family members do not know this information, care-givers can try the music that was popular during the resident's young adult years (Gibbons, 1977). Music preferred by staff, especially if the resident responds to it with cries, tensed muscles, and pained facial affect, must never be used in a resident's room unless it can be established that the resident also likes it.

Music must be used with caution because it can become tiresome to individuals who cannot turn it off when they no longer want to hear it. To have the best stimulative effect, music must be managed on a schedule (e.g., 15–20 minutes of music every hour may be adequate for some residents, whereas 1 hour of music followed by 1 hour of quiet time may be better for other residents). The schedule for each resident can be determined by noting resident responses to the use of music and by noting resident sleep patterns. Music is most appropriately played during the waking hours of the day or night.

Whether it is recorded or live, music can effectively elicit observable responses (e.g., changing facial expression and tension, increasing eye contact, vocal activity, and physical movements of arms, legs, and feet) in people with late-stage dementia (Cevasco & Grant, 2006; Clair, 1996; Sung & Chang, 2005). However, these manifestations of attentive behaviors do not occur in the same way in all people. Subjects (N = 26) in Clair's (1996) study of responses to singing as compared to reading the newspaper and silence fell into three behavioral categories: (1) people who seemed alert but were nonverbal and unresponsive, (2) people who seemed agitated as indicated by vocal activity and head turning, and (3) people who did not seem to be alert and were not generally responsive. The data for the 30-minute sessions held once a day for four consecutive days revealed that people in the first category exhibited significantly more facial responses to singing and reading than did subjects in other categories. The responses to singing were greater than they were for reading, but the difference was not statistically significant. It was postulated that perhaps the singing was more effective in the more alert people because they had demonstrated patterns of responding to stimuli in their environments even before the study began. Therefore, they may have been more open or more able to respond when vocal stimuli were presented. Some of these people seemed to sing along, changing pitches as the experimenter sang to them, although the melodies were not accurate and the words were not discernible. Other subjects may have closed down their ability to respond and may not have been able to access it in the short time the study ran. In addition, these subjects may have required more stimuli to interrupt the behaviors that were so integral to their daily lives. They may not have been willing or able to allow intrusion, at least for the time in which the stimuli were offered. With more stimuli over a longer time period, these persons may exhibit additional responses.

Observations reveal that singing familiar songs of youth without accompaniment effectively elicits positive responses in many people with late-stage dementia, whereas lullabies or the childhood chant "Na, na, na, na, na" is more effective with other people (Clair, 1996). This effectiveness is evident in changes in facial expression in people who are generally unresponsive, or it may be evident in the now-relaxed facial expressions of people who were agitated when the singing began, as indicated by their repetitive movements, jerking, or vocal activity, including screaming. In addition, singing a lullaby can calm and quiet people who moan or cry, at least temporarily.

Although many people with dementia are relaxed by singing, others respond vocally. Their vocal responses appear to be attempts to join in the singing, as in the following:

> Mr. Dahne, who had begun music therapy sessions in middle-stage dementia and was now in late-stage dementia, could no longer sing the lyrics or melodies of songs. However, he did

consistently make vocal responses in the same phrase of a familiar song each time it was sung to him.

Miss Tolliver, who screamed and cried during the day, gradually calmed when a music therapist sang to her. During each 30-minute music therapy session, Miss Tolliver's shrill, high-pitched, rapid vocalizations changed to a singsong type of vocalization, with lower pitch and slower articulations. Her rigid facial expressions relaxed, and she lowered her shoulders and smiled. Miss Tolliver seemed comforted as long as the singing continued.

Singing may be a particularly useful approach for people with dementia because it provides a point of contact with another human being and makes no cognitive demands. It may be associated with positive experiences and people, including parents or other nurturers who sang to and held individuals with dementia as children to calm and comfort them, throughout life. Singing directly to people and in proximity to them, even if they do not join in, can be beneficial. Singing can elicit positive responses when other resources are not available, and it requires no music training or equipment. It also is a way for family members and spouses to continue some interaction with a loved one.

Talking to individuals in late-stage dementia is also important as an effort to acknowledge them. Although they may not respond, they may be aware that someone is taking the time to offer them attention and to provide for their need to be with another person. Caregivers can talk about what is happening in the community, in their lives, or in the lives of others. The topic is not important, but it is essential that the discussion be directed toward the individual with dementia and that the conversation be structured as if the person with dementia comprehends everything. Issues that would not be discussed in the person's presence were he or she fully cognizant should not be discussed. Derogatory references to the individual's condition, expressions of deep pity for the person's inability to function, or other demeaning or possibly provocative comments should never be included in the conversation. Offering empathy in a soothing speaking voice or taking the time to read poetry, a story, or a newspaper article is often a touching gesture. The sound of a familiar voice may provide more comfort than a caregiver may be aware.

Singing or talking combined with touching can provide an even deeper level of human contact for people with late-stage dementia. Touching can include holding hands, hugging, holding and rocking, sitting in close proximity, placing an arm about the shoulders, gently stroking the brow or cheek, kissing, and caressing the face. Gentle massage using skin-conditioning creams or oils can provide satisfying responses and relief of tension. Whatever stimulation is provided, care must be taken to ensure its desirability. If muscles are relaxed and accompanied by facial expressions that are neutral or even pleasant, the stimuli is appropriate. However, if the person makes any effort to pull away, tense muscles in the face or body, turn the head away, or vocally respond in distress, the stimuli must be discontinued. The caregiver or therapist must listen with eyes, ears, heart, and hands to know how to appropriately approach individuals who cannot articulate their desires.

CONCLUSION

Music therapists design and implement programs that promote cooperative interaction and engagement in purposeful activities using music. Music therapy provides ways for family members to reintegrate a loved one with dementia into a family activity, for spouses to interact as a couple even if it is just for a short time, and for people with dementia to interact with others. These music therapy interventions are based on individual assessment of skills and abilities, designed to suit the individual response levels of people with dementia and their loved ones in order to allow them to participate, evaluated regularly to determine whether adjustments are needed, and altered as required to facilitate the best possible outcomes. These participants do not need a background or training in music in order for them to successfully involve themselves in applications such as rhythm playing, singing, and moving to music (Ebberts, 1994).

Some therapeutic interventions with music may be implemented by people who are not music therapists, provided they have the skills, abilities, and training to use them appropriately. It is feasible for a music therapist to work as a staff member or as a consultant, providing direct services to people with dementia, and to teach nursing staff, family members, or spouses to use music throughout the day to interact with people with dementia. Music therapists can also conduct training programs to guide caregivers in their efforts to provide care recipients with structure, opportunities for success and belonging, and quality of life throughout the stages of dementia. With the assistance of a music therapist and appropriate applications of music media, the quality of life of people with dementia can be enhanced and extended. Through music, they can continue to belong and to interact with others, to be part of a family, and to function at the highest level possible for them until they die. With music, they are not alone and their families can still touch them.

REFERENCES

Aldridge, A. (1995). Music therapy and the treatment of Alzheimer's disease. *Clinical Gerontologist*, 16(1), 41–57.

Aldridge, D. (2000). *Music therapy in dementia care*. London: Jessica Kingsley.

Anderson, M. A., Beaver, K. W., & Culliton, K. R. (Eds.). (1996). *The long-term care nursing assistant training manual* (2nd ed.). Baltimore: Health Professions Press.

Aneshensel, C. S., Pearlin, L. I., Levy-Storms, L., & Schuler, R. H. (2000). The transition from home to nursing home mortality among people with dementia. *The Journals of Gerontology Series B: Psychological Sciences and Social Sciences*, 55(3), S152–162.

Ashida, S. (2000). The effect of reminiscence music therapy sessions on changes in depressive symptoms in elderly persons with dementia. *Journal of Music Therapy*, 37(3), 170–182.

Beatty, W., Zavadil, K., Bailly, R., Rixen, G., Zavadil, L., Farnham, N., & Fisher, L. (1988). Preserved musical skill in a severely demented patient. *International Journal of Clinical Neuro-psychology*, 10(4), 158–164.

Bright, R. (1981). *Practical planning in music therapy for the aged*. Lynbrook, NY: Musicgraphics.

Bright, R. (1988). *Music therapy and the dementias: Improving the quality of life*. St. Louis, MO: MMB Music.

Bright, R. (1992). Music therapy in the management of dementia. In G. M. Jones & B. M. Miesen (Eds.), *Caregiving in dementia: Research and applications* (pp. 162–180). New York: Routledge.

Brotons, M. (2000). Overview of the music literature relating to elderly people. In D. Aldridge (Ed.), *Music therapy in dementia care* (pp. 33–62). London: Jessica Kingsley.

Brotons, M., & Pickett-Cooper, P. (1994). Preferences of Alzheimer's disease patients for music activities: Singing, instruments, dance/movement, games, and composition/improvisation. *Journal of Music Therapy*, 31(3), 220–233.

Cevasco, A. M., & Grant, R. E. (2006). Value of musical instruments used by the therapist to elicit responses from individuals in various stages of Alzheimer's disease. *Journal of Music Therapy*, 43(3), 226–246.

Chavin, M. (1991). *The lost chord: Reaching the person with dementia through the power of music.* Mt. Airy, MD: ElderSong Publications.

Christie, M. E. (1992). Music therapy applications in a skilled and intermediate care nursing home facility: A clinical study. *Activities, Adaptations, & Aging*, 16(4), 69–87.

Clair, A. A. (1991). Music therapy for severely regressed persons with probable diagnosis of Alzheimer's disease. In K. Bruscia (Ed.), *Case studies in music therapy* (pp. 571–580). Phoenixville, PA: Barcelona.

Clair, A. A. (2002). The effect of caregiver implemented music applications on mutual engagement in caregiver and care receiver couples with dementia. *The American Journal of Alzheimer's Disease & Other Dementias*, 17(5), 286–290.

Clair, A. A. (1996). Alert responses to singing stimuli in institutionalized persons with late stage dementia. *Journal of Music Therapy*, 33(4), 234–247.

Clair, A. A., & Bernstein, B. (1989). *A caregiver's guide to using music with persons who have severe dementia: An intro--*

duction. Unpublished manuscript, Colmery-O'Neil Veterans Affairs Medical Center, Topeka, KS.

Clair, A. A., & Bernstein, B. (1990a). A comparison of singing, vibrotactile and nonvibrotactile instrumental playing responses in severely regressed persons with dementia of the Alzheimer's type. *Journal of Music Therapy*, 27(3), 119–125.

Clair, A. A., & Bernstein, B. (1990b). A preliminary study of music therapy programming for severely regressed persons with Alzheimer's type dementia. *Journal of Applied Gerontology*, 9(3), 299–311.

Clair, A. A., & Bernstein, B. (1993). The preference for vibrotactile versus auditory stimuli in severely regressed persons with dementia of the Alzheimer's type compared with dementia due to ethanol abuse. *Music Therapy Perspectives*, 11(1), 24–27.

Clair, A. A., Bernstein, B., & Johnson, G. (1995). Rhythm characteristics in persons diagnosed with dementia, including those with probable Alzheimer's type. *Journal of Music Therapy*, 32(2), 113–131.

Clair, A. A., & Ebberts, A. G. (1997). The effects of music therapy on interactions between family caregivers and their care receivers with late stage dementia. *Journal of Music Therapy*, 34(3), 148–164.

Clair, A. A., Tebb, S., & Bernstein, B. (1993, January/February). The effects of a socialization and music therapy intervention on self-esteem and loneliness in spouse caregivers of those diagnosed with dementia of the Alzheimer's type: A pilot study. *American Journal of Alzheimer's Disease and Related Disorders and Research*, pp. 24–32.

Cuddy, L. L., & Duffin, J. (2005). Music, memory, and Alzheimer's disease: Is music recognition spared in dementia, and how can it be assessed? *Medical Hypotheses*, 64(2), 229–235.

Dementia: What are the common signs? (2003). *American Family Physician*, 67(5), 1051–1052.

Douglass, D. (1985). *Accent on rhythm: Music activities for the aged* (3rd ed.). St. Louis, MO: MMB Music.

Ebberts, A. (1994). *A comparison of the effects of movement with music, singing, and drumming on duration of engagement in care home residents who have late stage dementia.* Unpublished masters thesis, University of Kansas, Lawrence.

Edland, S. D., Roeca, W. A., Peterson, R. C., Cha, R. H., & Kokmen, E. (2002). Dementia and Alzheimer disease incidence rates do not vary by sex in Rochester, Minn. *Archives of Neurology*, 59(10), 1589–1593.

Feil, N. (1993). *The validation breakthrough: Simple techniques for communicating with people with "Alzheimer's-type dementia"* (pp. 27–28). Baltimore: Health Professions Press.

Finkel, S., Costa, E., Silva, J., Cohen, G., Miller, S., & Sartorius, N. (1996). Behavioral and psychological signs and symptoms of dementia: A consensus statement on current knowledge and implications for research and treatment. *International Psychogeriatrics*, 8(Suppl. 3), 497–500.

Gatz, J. L., Tyas, S. L., St. John, P., & Montgomery, P. (2005). Do depressive symptoms predict Alzheimer's disease and dementia? *The Journals of Gerontology Series: A Biological Sciences and Medical Sciences*, 60(6), 744–747.

Gfeller, K., & Hanson, N. (Eds.). (1995). *Music therapy programming for individuals with Alzheimer's disease and related disorders.* Iowa City: University of Iowa, College of Liberal Arts and College of Nursing.

Gibbons, A. C. (1977). Popular music preferences of elderly people. *Journal of Music Therapy*, 14(4), 180–189.

Gotell, E., Brown, S., & Ekman, S. L. (2000). Caregiver-assisted music events in psychogeriatric care. *Journal of Psychiatric and Mental Health Nursing*, 7(2), 119–125.

Groene, R. (2001). The effect of presentation and accompaniment styles on attentional and responsive behaviors of participants with dementia diagnoses. *Journal of Music Therapy*, 38(1), 36–50.

Groene, R. (1993). Effectiveness of music therapy 1:1 intervention with individuals having senile dementia of the Alzheimer's type. *Journal of Music Therapy*, 30(3), 138–157.

Hanser, S. S. (1990). A music therapy strategy for depressed older adults in the community. *Journal of Applied Gerontology*, 9(3), 283–298.

Hart, M. (1990). *Drumming at the edge of magic*. New York: Harper Collins.

Hebert, L. E., Scherr, P. A., Bienias, J. L., Bennett, D. A., & Evans, D. A. (2003). Alzheimer disease in the U.S. population: Prevalence estimates using the 2000 census. *Archives of Neurology*, 60(8), 1119–1122.

Hendrie, H. C. (1998). Epidemiology of dementia and Alzheimer's disease. *The American Journal of Geriatric Psychiatry*, 6(2 Suppl. 1), S3–18.

Iliffe, S., Manthorpe, J., & Eden, J. (2003). Sooner or later? Issues in the early diagnosis of dementia in general practice: A qualitative study. *Family Practice*, 20(4), 376–381.

Kales, H. C., Blow, F. C., Copeland, L. A., Bingham, R. C., Kammerer, E. E., & Mellow, A. M. (1999). Health care utilization by older patients with coexisting dementia and depression. *American Journal of Psychiatry*, 156(4), 550–556.

Knopman, D. S., Berg, J. D., Thomas, R., Grundman, M., Thal, L. J., & Sano, M. (1999). Nursing home placement is related to dementia progression: Experience from a clinical trial: Alzheimer's Disease Cooperative Study. *Neurology*, 5(4), 714–718.

Lipe, A. W. (1991). Using music therapy to enhance the quality of life in a client with Alzheimer's dementia: A case study. *Music Therapy Perspectives*, 9, 102–105.

Lucero, M. (1995). *Creative interventions with Alzheimer's patients*. Workshop sponsored by Manor HealthCare, the Topeka Alzheimer's Association, and Stormont-Vail Regional Medical Center, Topeka, KS.

Lynch, L. (1987). Music therapy: Its historical relationships and value in programs for the long-term care setting. In B. Karras (Ed.), *You bring out the music in me: Music in nursing homes* (pp. 5–16). New York: Haworth Press.

Moore, R. S., Staum, M. J., & Brotons, M. (1992). Music preferences of the elderly: Repertoire, vocal ranges, tempos, and accompaniments for singing. *Journal of Music Therapy*, 29(4), 236–252.

Olderog Millard, K. A., & Smith, J. M. (1989). The influence of group singing therapy on the behavior of Alzheimer's disease patients. *Journal of Music Therapy*, 26(2), 58–70.

Omnibus Budget Reconciliation Act of 1987. (1987). 100th Congress, First Session, Pub. L. No. 100-203. Washington, DC: U.S. Government Printing Office.

Palo-Bengtsson, L., & Ekman, S. L. (2000). Dance events as a caregiver intervention for persons with dementia. *Nursing Inquiry*, 7(3), 156–165.

Palo-Bengtsson, L., Winblad, B., Ekman, S. L. (1998). Social dancing: A way to support intellectual, emotional and motor functions in persons with dementia. *Journal of Psychiatric and Mental Health Nursing*, 5(6), 545–554.

Pollack, N., & Namazi, K. (1992). The effect of music participation on the social behavior of Alzheimer's disease patients. *Journal of Music Therapy*, 29(1), 54–67.

Prickett, C., & Moore, R. (1991). The use of music to aid memory of Alzheimer's patients. *Journal of Music Therapy*, 28(2), 101–110.

Ringman, J. M., & Cummings, J. L. (2006). Current and emerging pharmacological treatment options for dementia. *Behavioral Neurology*, 17(1), 5–16.

Reisberg, B., Ferris, S., & Franssen, E. (1985). An ordinal functional assessment tool for Alzheimer's type dementia. *Hospital Community Psychiatry*, 36(6), 593–595.

Ridder, H. M. O., & Aldridge, D. (2005). Individual music therapy for persons with frontotemporal dementia: Singing dialogue. *Nordic Journal of Music Therapy*, 14(2), 91–106.

Rules and Regulations 48871. *Requirements for long term care facilities*, 56 Fed. Reg. 187, 483.15(a). (1991).

Savundranayagam, M. V., Hummert, M. L., & Montgomery, R. J. V. (2005). Investigating the effects of communication problems on problems of caregiver burden. *The Journals of Gerontology Series B: Psychological Sciences and Social Sciences*, 60(1), S48–S55.

Shaw, J. (1993). *The joy of music in maturity*. St. Louis, MO: MMB Music.

Sixsmith, A., & Gibson, G. (2006). Music and the wellbeing of people with dementia. *Aging and Society*, 27(1), 127–145.

Smith, G. E., Kokmen, E., & O'Brien, P. C. (2000). Risk factors for nursing home placement in a population-based dementia cohort. *Journal of the American Geriatrics Society*, 48(5), 519–525.

Snyder, L., Jenkins, C., & Joosten, L. (2007). Effectiveness of support groups for people with mild to moderate Alzheimer's disease: An evaluative survey. *American Journal of Alzheimer's Disease and Other Dementias*, 22(1), 14–19.

Sung, H., & Chang, A. M. (2005). Use of preferred music to decrease agitated behaviours in older people with dementia: A review of the literature. *Journal of Clinical Nursing*, 14(9), 1133–1140.

Takahashi, T., & Matsushita, H. (2006). Long-term effects of music therapy on elderly with moderate/severe dementia. *Journal of Music Therapy*, 43(4), 317–333.

Voelkl, J., Fries, B., & Galecki, A. (1995). Predictors of nursing home residents' participation in activity programs. *Gerontologist*, 35(1), 44–51.

Whitcomb, J. (1989, July/August). Thanks for the memory. *American Journal of Alzheimer's Care and Related Disorders and Research*, pp. 22–33.

Whitcomb, J. (1993, Spring). Will you love me in December? *Connections*, pp. 8–9, 14–15.

Whitehouse, P. (1992). Dementia: The medical perspective. In R. H. Binstock, S. G. Post, & P. J. Whitehouse (Eds.), *Dementia and aging: Ethics, values, and policy choices* (pp. 21–29). Baltimore: The Johns Hopkins University Press.

Zarit, S. H., Femia, E. E., Watson, J., Rice-Oeschger, L., & Kakos, B. (2004). Memory club: A group intervention for people with early-stage dementia and their care partners. *The Gerontologist*, 44(2), 262–269.

Chapter 4

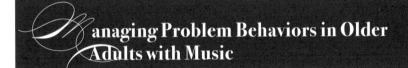

Managing Problem Behaviors in Older Adults with Music

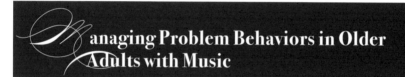

Managing Problem Behaviors in Older Adults with Music

Some older people display behaviors that are harmful to their own health and well-being as well as that of their caregivers. These behaviors are associated with the physical frailties and emotional stresses that accompany normal aging and with progressive dementia. Problem behaviors include, but are not limited to, depression, insomnia, agitation, inability to perform activities of daily living (ADLs), and catastrophic reactions.

DEPRESSION

Depression is a mood disorder that can range from mild to severe, wherein psychotic features may be present (American Psychiatric Association [APA], 2000). Depression may be a response to bereavement (Twedell & O'Neil, 2007), a result of medical conditions or substance abuse, a reaction to medications or toxins, or a manifestation of dementia (APA, 2000). It may be difficult to determine whether symptoms are the result of depression or dementia. In depressed people, the decline of memory and intellectual abilities is usually recent, has a rapid progression, and can be described in accurate detail by depressed individuals (Ropper & Brown, 2005). Furthermore, people with dementia attempt to hide their confusion and deny their memory losses, whereas depressed people readily admit the same symptoms (Lucero, 1995).

To make a diagnosis of depression, a clinician must determine that five or more symptoms of depression are present. These symptoms must include either depressed mood or loss of interest or pleasure in activities previously enjoyed, combined with weight gain or loss, insomnia or hypersomnia, psychomotor agitation or retardation, fatigue or loss of energy, feelings of worthlessness or guilt, inability to concentrate, and recurrent thoughts of death (APA, 2000). Suicidal ideation (thinking about committing suicide) and suicide are serious consequences of depression. Suicidal thoughts occur in 4 out of every 5 depressed people, with 3 of 5 people seriously considering suicide (Sadock & Sadock, 2004).

Because of the serious nature of depression and its harmful consequences, it is essential that depressed people seek treatment. If pharmacological management (antidepressant medication) is indicated, responses to the medication must be monitored carefully and any adverse effects reported immediately to the physician in charge. Although medical intervention is effective in treating depression in older people, it takes 4–6 weeks for nearly all antidepressants to become established in the bloodstream. Consequently, there is a need for vigilance, support, and encouragement during the treatment process (Isselbacher, Braunwald, Wilson, Martin, Fauci, & Kasper, 1994). Harmful effects can be avoided by careful monitoring of the effects of treatment and by feedback to physicians, who can adjust dosages and types of medication.

Music Intervention

Used in conjunction with medical intervention, music therapy may help relieve the symptoms of depression. Hanser (1990) studied a group of four individuals diagnosed with depression who ranged in age from 65 to 74 years and who used music with relaxation techniques to reduce anxiety and depressive symptoms. Hanser offered each person an opportunity to select the music he or she preferred and a relaxation technique that was the most practical to use at home. The techniques available using music in relaxation included the following:

1. Gentle exercise while listening to familiar music that has positive associations

2. Facial muscle self-massage while listening to enjoyable music

3. Progressive muscle relaxation with deep breathing while listening to music

4. Guided imagery (see Chapter 5) with music to replace depressing or anxious thought

5. Imagery while using music that alleviated discomfort associate with depression or anxiety.

After teaching each person to use his or her chosen technique, she asked that it be practiced regularly. She monitored all relaxation approaches once each week and provided assistance when needed. After 8 weeks, each person reported a decrease in anxiety, somatic complaints, and self-perceived levels of depression.

Using music to relax or to alleviate physical discomfort empowers people to manage their quality of life and may relieve some of the symptoms of depression that are associated with illness and disability. It is essential for people to choose the music that is most effective for them and that agrees with their tastes and preferences. It is also important to guard against using music recklessly in imagery.

Guided Imagery and Music (see Chapter 5) requires many hours of training and supervision in order to help people cope with the issues that surface when they are relaxed while listening to music (Summer, 1990). This training includes developing the skills necessary to use music to induce imagery experiences, to process the material that surfaces in imagery, and to select the appropriate music for all components of the experience. When people without skills training experiment with music and images, associations and memories that lead to distress can be tapped unexpectedly. Although some associations and memories are pleasant and give no cause for alarm, others can cause harmful reactions. Unresolved memories of events or behaviors that were emotionally and/or physically painful can surface suddenly when people are relaxed and defenseless. These events or behaviors can contribute to the feelings of depression, particularly if there is no way to resolve them.

One way to use music to relieve depression is to incorporate progressively more stimulating music. The exercise begins with music that matches the mood of the individual. If the person feels somber, depressed, and unmotivated, the music begins with a very slow tempo and a minor tonality. The music sounds sad and is characterized by unaccented and unsyncopated beats. When selecting a slow, sad piece of music for an individual, it is particularly helpful if the tempo of the music matches the individual's rate of breathing. The selection is played and the person is asked to breathe with it. When the music concludes, the next selection is introduced.

The second selection has a slightly faster tempo, but the beats are unaccented and unsyncopated, with minor tonality. The second selection is also played for several minutes, and the individual is again asked to breathe with the music. This piece must be played long enough to allow the individual's breathing to become closely synchronized with the rhythm. If synchrony does not occur, but the breathing is deeper than it was at the beginning of the first selection, it is time to move on to the third piece of music.

The third musical selection has a slightly quicker tempo and it may have a major tonality. Again, the individual is directed to listen to the music and to tap a toe or a finger to it. Some simple exercises may be introduced at this point, provided the person is physically able to participate. If the person wishes to exercise, he or she is directed to place a hand behind the head with the elbow on a plane parallel to the shoulder. Then the individual is instructed to raise the hand while extending the arm up and out as far as possible from the body. The arm movements continue up and back in time to the music while mimicking the instructor's movements and following the counts (e.g., "Up 2, 3, 4; down, 2, 3, 4"). The regimen is repeated for as many as eight repetitions for each arm, or for as long as the person can tolerate the arm movements. After several repetitions, the person can be directed to rest the arm movements while continuing to focus on a breathing pattern that forces the carbon dioxide from the lungs. This breathing pattern requires an inhalation followed by an exhalation requiring twice the time used in the inhalation. Other exercise arm movements during the breathing pattern are optional. Repeating the breathing pattern in time to the music increases oxygen intake and heart rate, and these increases can lift, at least temporarily, the depressed mood (Thaut, 2002).

Once a person is moving to the music while breathing with lengthened exhalation, the fourth musical selection can be introduced. The tempo is slightly faster than the third selection, and accented beats with syncopation are recommended. The person is encouraged to move in time to the music. If the individual must remain seated, he or she can move feet and legs in time to the music or can sway back and forth while moving arms in time to the beat. After several minutes of movement with this fast-paced, stimulative music, facial expressions may be pleasant, shoulders may be more erect and less slumped, and breathing may be less shallow than before the music intervention was introduced.

A progressively more stimulative music program, such as the one described here, can be practiced every day and can be repeated within the course of a day. Depressed people are not motivated to participate in many activities, and it may be difficult to encourage them to make the effort, at least initially. However, music may facilitate their subsequent involvement.

Although progressively more stimulating music increases motor activity and physical responses by increasing the heart rate and improving the oxygen exchange during respiration, the most pleasant and active responses are generated by preferred music, music that carries with it fond memories and associations. The use of high-quality recordings of this music played at a volume that older people can hear easily produces these responses.

INSOMNIA

Insomnia is characterized by difficulty falling asleep, inability to fall asleep, and wakefulness during sleep, which can lead to the inappropriate use of medications (e.g., hypnotics or alcohol to facilitate sleep, anxiolytics to decrease anxiety or tension, caffeine or other stimulants to combat fatigue) (APA, 2000). Although alcohol increases drowsiness and decreases the time required to fall asleep, moderate amounts of alcohol increase the number of intermittent awakenings by interfering with the brain's ability to maintain sleep. In addition, caffeine prolongs the period before sleep, causes more frequent arousals during sleep, and reduces total sleep time for as long as 8–14 hours after ingestion (Kasper, Braunwald, Fauci, Hauser, Longo, & Jameson, 2004). Complaints of insomnia are more common among older people, although they are more likely to experience difficulty maintaining sleep and to experience early morning awakenings than they are to have difficulty falling asleep (APA, 2000).

Often people experience insomnia when they are in an unfamiliar environment, such as a hotel or a hospital room, or when they experience or anticipate a traumatic, stressful, or exciting event; a time change; an illness; or an injury. Although inadequate sleep may be transient, short-term, or long-term, persistent insomnia can impair daytime functioning, disturb moods, and increase the risk of accident-related injury (Kasper et al., 2004). Lack of sleep can impair responsiveness, sap energy, dull the cognitive processes, increase moodiness, impede tolerance of others, and generally decrease feelings of well-being. It is therefore essential to determine the cause of insomnia and identify an appropriate intervention.

Insomnia can result from a number of causes, and a thorough medical examination is indicated if sleeplessness occurs for any extended period of time. Once the cause is determined, recommended interventions may include medication, exercise, and relaxation techniques.

Music Intervention in Insomnia

Music can be used to enhance the effects of relaxation that promote sleep. Hanser (1990) designed music therapy applications to decrease insomnia in four depressed people. She recommended the daily practice of individually selected relaxation techniques with music. She argued that practicing at times when stress was low provided the opportunity to learn and fully grasp how to use the technique. Then, as individuals became familiar with the feelings of relaxation associated with the technique and the music, they could successfully use the technique and music when relaxation was desired. Once they learned to relax using their music, they were asked to listen to the music at bedtime. Because the music was associated with practiced relaxation responses, it relaxed them when they heard it before going to sleep.

In order to implement a relaxation technique at bedtime, it is important to use sound equipment that automatically shuts off so that it is not necessary to manually control it once sleep is induced. It is also important that this equipment is of sufficient quality to avoid distortion or other distractions, and the person using it must consider whether a roommate or spouse would find the music disturbing. If so, some arrangement may be made to use headphones or an ear jack. However, these devices have certain disadvantages. They may disturb sleep if the head is turned, and if they are removed by someone in attendance, he or she may awaken a person who has struggled to go to sleep. Therefore, free field presentation of the music at a volume sufficient to mask other environmental sounds is best.

It is also best to use a recording of the music with which the person has practiced and has familiarity. This familiarity tends to induce inattention and drowsiness, provided the individual has not slept for hours. Any new or unfamiliar music is a novelty, which raises the attention level, and music on the radio is distracting because it is periodically interrupted by spoken commentary or advertisements. The music that has been selected to aid in sleep must have qualities that promote sleep. It should have no sudden or dramatic changes in tempo, volume, or rhythm; it should be nonpercussive with no syncopation; and it should have a tempo that is slow enough to promote relaxation rather than movement.

To begin the relaxation technique, a person should lie in bed and adjust his or her bedclothes for comfort. The music should be turned on and the lights turned off. The individual should empty his or her mind of all thoughts and concerns. The person may find it difficult at first. If the person is receptive, a technique that has helped many people is the following guided experience:

> Picture yourself standing or sitting on the shore of a stream as a boat comes into view. As the boat floats by you, place all your thoughts on it and watch them float away. When other thoughts come to you, place them on another boat and watch them float away. Do this until all your thoughts have floated away. (Dossey, 1993, p. 29)

The person is now ready to implement his or her relaxation technique.

Individuals must place themselves (or be placed) on a sleep regimen that includes preparation time. Preparation time is a preplanned amount of time during which a person decreases his or her activities before attempting to sleep. During this time, it may be helpful for the individual to separate from involvement with other people and begin to let go of the cares and concerns of the day. Time spent reading, listening to a book, or watching videos or television programs that are pleasant and calming can also be helpful. To further encourage sleep, a regular sleep schedule and a specific place to sleep must be determined. Individuals must avoid naps, and activities other than sleeping must not take place in bed (e.g., eating snacks or meals, reading, lounging, watching television).

A careful survey of the sleep environment may reveal reasons for disruptions in sleep. The temperature of the room may be either too warm or too cool to promote sleep, bedclothes may be uncomfortable, lighting may emit disturbing low- or high-frequency sounds, neighborhood dogs and cats may make noise, a luminous clock dial may clearly show the duration of wakefulness, or a spouse or room-mate may be restless. Such difficulties must be resolved in order for sleep to be satisfactory.

AGITATION

Agitation refers to a range of behaviors that are judged by an observer to be inappropriate verbalizations, vocalizations, or motor activities such as pacing or wandering that has no apparent purpose (Cohen-Mansfield, 1986; Spira & Edelstein, 2006). (*Inappropriate* may be defined as abusiveness and aggressiveness and the frequency thereof, and the relationship of the behavior to accepted social stan-dards.) Agitation may be manifested by pacing, moving furniture, or relocating objects. These activities may or may not be accompanied by verbalizations or vocalizations that may be irritating or even offen-sive to other people. Agitation may be caused by anger, depression, anxiety, restlessness, boredom, medication, or dementia (Mace & Rabins, 1999). Lucero (1995) indicated that the agitation displayed by people with late-stage dementia may be the result of pain and dis-comfort. Therefore, pain medication is indicated when other forms of treatment have had little or no effect.

To effectively ameliorate the symptoms of agitation, the cause must be ascertained. Consultation with a geriatrician is indicated when symptoms persist, but much dementia-related agitation can be diminished using a predictable routine in a structured environment that allows individuals the freedom to move about. Predictability and structure provide order for people who are confused and who can-not organize for themselves. These qualities tend to calm people who would otherwise be agitated in environments that are constantly changing.

Music Intervention in Agitation

Music provides structure and predictability through its rhythm, form, and familiarity. One beat follows the next in music, and people with dementia can easily follow a rhythmic pulse whether embedded in music or played only on percussion instruments. Familiar songs from the past offer people with dementia opportunities to participate in singing, dancing/moving to the music, or playing a rhythmic accompaniment. Such participation facilitates mental organization and allows people with dementia to respond meaningfully to sensory stimulation (Thaut, 2002).

A research study of 24 people diagnosed with late-stage dementia who regularly exhibited agitated behaviors showed that they could engage effectively in music therapy. When the subjects were compared for duration of participation in singing, movement, and drumming, they participated longer in both movement and drumming than they did in singing. No significant difference was observed between participation in drumming and participation in movement. Therefore, evidence exists that agitated people with late-stage dementia can respond positively to structured music interventions (Ebberts, 1994). A separate case study also described music as a viable intervention to decrease wandering and induce engagement in people with dementia (Fitzgerald-Cloutier, 1993).

Although there is evidence that playing percussion instruments (e.g., drums) and moving in time to music yield positive results, preferences for music and types of participation in music may vary from person to person. Some people respond immediately to songs from their young adult years, whereas others respond to songs from their childhood. Certain individuals respond quickly to music that causes them to clap their hands or tap their feet in time with the music, whereas others may respond best to the dance music of their young adult years, which causes them to dance or to play percussion instruments.

Whatever type of participation is preferred, the music used for it must begin with a tempo that is commensurate with individual physical and emotional activity levels. The physical behaviors of agitation are characterized by rapid movement. Individuals may remain in one place and confine their movements to rapidly rocking back and forth. Other agitated people may ambulate, quickly pacing around a particular area or up and down a hallway. Emotional outbursts may accompany these physical behaviors and are usually manifested by vocalizations or verbalizations, such as shrieks, cries, or screams. The tempo of the music is matched to individuals' physical movements and the volume is adjusted so that it can be heard. The music must also be portable to move with certain individuals (e.g., agitated people who pace).

Because the pace and the volume of the music must be readily adjusted to the physical movements of the agitated individuals, generally it must be performed live. Caregivers can sing to care recipients while walking beside them or facing them, if possible. They may take one or both hands in their own and swing the individual's arms in time to the music and move with them. If an individual stops pacing, the caregiver can swing both arms in time to the music. By using songs such as "Down by the Riverside," "When the Saints Go Marchin' In," or "Home on the Range," which the care recipient likely knows through background and experience, caregivers can provide a context that the care recipient recognizes as pleasant and familiar. Familiarity provides predictability and the structure of the music provides security of that which is known and understood on some level.

As the caregiver continues to elicit responses from the care recipient, the volume of the music can be decreased and the tempo can be slowed. As quieter music and slower movements become possible, the care recipient is likely to relax further, as indicated by lowering the shoulders, relaxing the wrinkles in the forehead, and raising, rather than knitting, the eyebrows. When the individual does not respond to the stimuli and he or she continues to be agitated, the caregiver must remain active and the music must remain loud until the agitated person responds appropriately. Once the individual relaxes, it is possible to direct him or her to some other activity.

Although many agitated people respond to singing, others respond best to playing a percussion instrument. When an agitated person with this preference is pacing, the caregiver should walk alongside and hold out a drum mallet so the care recipient can easily grasp the handle. Then an easily held drum (e.g., paddle drum, frame drum) is handed to the individual. The care recipient will begin to hit the drum with the mallet almost immediately, particularly if the caregiver walking alongside also holds and hits a drum to model the behavior. The caregiver and the care recipient may walk side by side, playing their drums at a tempo and a volume that suits the agitated mood and the activity that results from it. The tempo and the volume may be decreased as the agitated mood begins to dissipate. The pace will slow until the individual is able to stand and face the caregiver while continuing to play the drum. The caregiver and the care recipient may interact using their instruments in a "call and response" pattern. Call and response is a pattern in which one person plays a fragment of melody or a rhythm pattern and the other person plays a fragment that is similar but differs in that it is a response to the first fragment. If the care recipient is calm enough to be able to engage in behavior at this level, then the agitated mood has passed, and the two individuals can engage in nonverbal interactions with music. For example, the caregiver may take both the mallet and the drum from the care recipient and move them out of the way. The caregiver may then face the care recipient, place his or her hands on the recipient's shoulders or upper arms, and sway with music. The music may be recorded or sung by the caregiver. While making eye contact, the caregiver and care recipient can move about the room or sway in place to the music. In general, people with dementia respond to this closeness with pleasant facial expressions and even smiles.

ACTIVITIES OF DAILY LIVING

ADLs (e.g., eating, bathing, dressing, toileting) are necessary for general health and personal comfort (Galasko, Schmidt, Thomas, Jin, Bennett, & Ferris, 2005). As some people age, they require assistance with some or all ADLs, depending on their ability to function. They may become too physically frail or too confused to perform ADLs. It is important to the care recipients' dignity, self-esteem, and maintenance of capabilities for caregivers to allow them to perform ADLs to the best of their ability. Helping older people perform ADLs may be more time-consuming than performing the ADLs for them. However, allowing sufficient time helps older individuals maintain their self-esteem and dignity. As a result, older people will be less of a care burden for their caregivers.

Agitation and resistance with ADLs may be due to sudden changes in participation requirements or in the environment that triggers stress responses. With insufficient cognitive function to understand the changes, the stress response of "fight or flight" (Selye, 1956) likely engages. Though stress responses and stress management are described more fully in Chapter 5, stress evoked during activity shifts in daily routines may be lessened or prevented by (1) play-ing recordings of familiar and preferred music just prior to an activity change, followed by (2) singing, rather than speaking, instructions for the task one step at a time. Without stress, persons are more likely to perform well-rehearsed, habitual activities such as dressing, toilet-ing, bathing, or eating.

Eating Problems

Assistance with eating for older people ranges from occa-sional prompts to place food on a utensil and then in their mouths, to step-by-step assistance with verbal and physical cues for each task required to eat a single bite. When eating ceases, as often happens in late-stage dementia, or when aspiration of food or liquid into the lungs cannot be ameliorated through rehabilitation following other severe neurological impairments such as those resulting from a stroke or Parkinson's disease, the implantation of a tube for gastrointestinal feeding is required.

People who can eat on their own may have serious problems with adequate nutrition and hydration because they become easily distracted, especially if they have dementia. They may require contin-ual reminders to take a bite, chew, and then swallow. A light touch on the elbow may trigger self-feeding in people who do not respond well to verbal reminders (Lucero, 1995). To encourage eating, a properly structured dining environment is essential. The following lists some approaches to proper structure:

- Eliminate noise and other stimuli that distract attention
- Place only one food on the plate at a time
- Adapt utensils for easy grasping
- Use plates with rims to help diners guide food onto utensils and plates with suction cups on the bottoms to prevent sliding
- Arrange seating so that compatible people arc seated together
- Maintain a routine that uses the same seating for each meal
- Provide verbal cues and physical prompts when needed
- Make sure preferred foods are served often
- Provide music because it rhythmically structures the environment as it provides familiarity and pleasant associations.

Even with appropriate environmental conditions, completing a well-balanced meal with the appropriate number of calories may require a lengthy time period. The proper nutrition of older people is a constant concern of caregivers because functioning to the fullest extent possible depends on it. People who wander or pace are of particular concern because they are physically active and therefore require even more calories to maintain their weight. Portable foods eaten with fingers while walking, in addition to regular and frequent meals, are recommended for these persons throughout the day. Without proper nutrition, illnesses are more common, infections occur more frequently, and care is more difficult and costly (Mathey, Vanneste, de Graaf, de Groot, & van Staveren, 2001).

Music Interventions in Eating Problems

Often, music is used to enhance the eating environments of long-term care facilities (Aldridge, 2007). Music establishes a positive mood, focuses attention, and stimulates response in some individuals with dementia. Therefore, it is important that the music be neither markedly sedative (because it can induce drowsiness and inactivity) nor markedly stimulative (because it can induce a need to stand up and move). The rhythm and tempo of the music must be conducive to activity while masking noise and other sounds that may divert attention from eating. Upbeat music with moderate, danceable tempos and familiar, singable melodies is most appropriate. The music that was popular in residents' young adult years tends to stimulate productive responses. Music that is unfamiliar or that is played in an unfamiliar style tends to disrupt eating and has other harmful effects, ranging from agitation to withdrawal. The volume of the music during dining may also be a factor in eating behaviors, but no information is available concerning appropriate volume. It seems that music played at a comfortable, audible level and on high-quality sound equipment (to avoid distortion that may stimulate agitation or inattention) is the most appropriate.

Music in the environment may attract persons who wander to come into the dining area and may help decrease or stop their pacing for a time. Even if these persons refuse to sit to eat, they may respond to food presented to them while in an environment where their preferred music is playing. The music may further help to engage them in established eating habits, particularly if they are provided with on-going prompts by one who is familiar with their usual eating patterns and food preferences, for example, using ketchup on meat and veg-etables to sweeten them.

Bathing, Dressing, and Toileting Problems

Assistance with bathing, dressing, and toileting ranges from providing verbal cues to physically performing these tasks. Skills deteriorate and increased confusion is apparent over time in people with progressive dementia. People with late-stage dementia also lose the ability to regulate body temperature, and rooms that are either too warm or too cool can cause people with dementia to become agitated, even aggressive (Lucero, 1995). They may become emotionally upset and agitated when their clothing is disturbed, and they may retaliate by physically striking their caregivers. Residents of care facilities may also become upset and agitated when they are approached by nursing staff, particularly if they do not recognize the face of a staff member or if they do not associate the staff member with positive experiences.

People with dementia also have difficulty toileting them-selves. They may have lost bowel and bladder control, may be too preoccupied to toilet themselves, or may not remember the location of the toilet. Caregivers work continuously to keep these individuals clean and dry. People who can still toilet themselves are reminded to use the toilet and are escorted to the toilet, if necessary. The cloth-ing of people who are incontinent is checked regularly and changed if necessary. (A two-hour schedule for toileting helps avoid soiling.) These efforts are integral to maintaining skin integrity, which keeps infection under control and subsequently contributes to good physi-cal health.

Music Interventions in Bathing, Dressing, and Toileting

To circumvent problem behavior in bathing, dressing, and toileting, caregivers may attempt to establish a secure environment by singing songs or playing music that is familiar or preferred to care re-cipients (Clark, Lipe & Bilbrey, 1998). Singing may provide access to feelings of comfort that are associated with times when they were nur-tured (e.g., when their mothers sang lullabies to comfort them when they were frightened or hurt, to quiet them when it was time to go to sleep) and with feelings of belonging. For example, many individuals bonded by singing together in school, in church, in expressions of patriotism, and during significant events.

The songs that are likely to be successful with confused care recipients were memorized early in life and are therefore readily accessible through long-term memory. Caregivers who sing to care recipients during ADLs will find that these older adults gradually become physically relaxed. They may observe changes in posture from tight, lifted shoulders with raised arms and clenched fists to lowered shoulders and lowered arms with unclenched hands; changes in facial expression from furrowed brows and tight jaws to smooth brows and relaxed jaws; and changes in vocal activity from loud, distressed vocal pleas and even screams or cries to quieter, more conversational vocalizations. Care recipients may even sing along or make vocalizations that indicate an attempt to sing.

Often, caregivers react to suggestions that they sing to their care recipients by saying, "I can't sing," or "I'm older now and my voice isn't as good as it used to be." These responses reflect a lack of confidence. Caregivers must be reassured that what is important is not the quality of the voice but the contact that singing provides with another human being and the connections it makes with any residual memory of positive experiences.

> Mrs. Roth was encouraged by a music therapist to sing to her husband who had dementia. Mrs. Roth said, "I just don't have a pretty singing voice." The music therapist was quick to reply, "You've been married to him for over 50 years. You have had a wonderfully satisfying relationship. So your voice is going to be the very best one he will ever hear, no matter how bad you think it is." Mrs. Roth thought for a moment and then said, "You know, he used to call me his 'little songbird' when we were newlyweds."

> Later that day Mrs. Roth confessed that she had sung to her husband when no one else was in his room at the residential care facility and that he had looked into her eyes. She felt pleased to have tried it and elicited a response from her husband.

CATASTROPHIC REACTIONS

Catastrophic reactions are displayed by people who are confused because of illness or by people with dementia. These behaviors do not appear to be signs of illness, but are perceived simply as obstinate, critical, or overly emotional behaviors (Mace & Rabins, 1999). The behaviors occur when people are no longer able to respond as they did before their illness. They may feel overwhelmed by simple tasks that require them to do several things at once (e.g., taking a bath is preceded by undressing, which involves unbuttoning buttons, unzipping zippers, slipping clothing over the head or down the legs, pulling off shoes and stockings before the tub is entered). Thus, they may respond to a request to take a bath by being stubborn and becoming increasingly upset until everyone is distraught.

Once an individual in a long-term care facility reacts catastrophically to a person or an event, similar responses may be triggered in other residents. The catastrophic behavior almost seems to set off a chain reaction. However, people likely react out of fear and confusion. The potential for physical injury and emotional trauma is great. Therefore, the best way to manage catastrophic behaviors is to avoid them whenever possible.

Catastrophic behavior may result from any activity, but usually some warning is given. For example, individuals become progressively animated, vocal, and even physically aggressive. If the warning is not heeded, the catastrophic behaviors can escalate beyond caregivers' control. Efforts to curb these behaviors are not usually successful and they increase the risk for physical injury to both the caregiver and the care recipient.

One of the warning signs of potentially catastrophic behaviors is resistance. People with dementia may resist following regimens, cooperating with others, or allowing others in close proximity. Some people resist because they do not understand what is being asked of them or because they want to exercise their abilities to set boundaries and have some control over their lives. As they grow more fragile and confused, there is little over which they can exercise control. When people with dementia resist, it is often effective to allow them this decision. Approaching them a few minutes later or even later in the day can often result in cooperation. However, the length of the delay depends on the task. If the task is administering medication on schedule or on putting dry, clean clothing, the delay must be short. However, if a person is scheduled for therapy and the time is flexible, there is no need to adhere to an exact schedule. The schedules and procedures that provide structure and reduce agitation in some older adults are the same schedules and procedures that deprive some people of the power to make their own decisions. Often, they are cooperative if time is taken to inform them of what is about to happen and to validate their concerns. Even people who do not appear to understand the information respond positively to others' efforts to acknowledge them as people and to be genuinely empathic to their situation. Language that is direct and economical and spoken in person using appropriate affect can be the most successful in persuading an individual to give permission to carry out procedures.

> Mrs. Ferdin was waiting for her music therapy session to begin. As she waited, she talked with a child who had come to visit his grandfather. Mrs. Ferdin seemed very invested in her conversation with the boy, speaking softly to him while she held his hand. Her expression was one of great pleasure. When the music therapist asked if she was ready to leave the boy and come to music therapy, Mrs. Ferdin's voice became loud and gruff, her brow furrowed, and her jaw clenched. She refused to leave the child and became combative with a staff member. The music therapist said that she understood she was not ready to come to therapy and that she would check with her later. When the therapist left her, Mrs. Ferdin resumed her conversation with the boy. The music therapist began to work with another resident who was willing to come to therapy at an earlier time. Upon completing the session, the music therapist went to find Mrs. Ferdin. She found her alone, the visit with the boy over. When asked if she would come to the music therapy session, Mrs. Ferdin smiled, held out her hand for the music therapist to hold, and accompanied her to the music therapy room.

Sometimes resistance occurs as the result of delusional thoughts with which the person is preoccupied. Feil and De Klerk-

Rubin (2002) attributed these delusional thoughts to unresolved business from the past and emphasized the need for caregivers and others to approach these people by validating them. Caregivers should ask their delusional care recipients about their thoughts and engage them in conversation about the thoughts, thereby validating them and fostering cooperation. Any discussion that attempts to discredit the delusional thoughts results in argument, which can quickly escalate to catastrophic proportions, such as physical combativeness, or to complete withdrawal. The following vignette demonstrates the successful use of validation with a person with dementia:

> Instead of walking to his music therapy session, Mr. Conley was walking down the hall, looking down at his feet as he placed one carefully in front of the other, heel to toe. When he was approached by his music therapist, Mrs. Bronway, he asked, "What are you doing up here?" She looked at him, puzzled. Mr. Conley said, "You know we're up on the 10th floor girders of this construction site. Be careful or you'll fall!" Mrs. Bronway said, "But it's time to go to your music therapy session." He countered, "I can't go anywhere. I'm on the job." She then asked, "Are you Union?" He replied, "Well, yes I am." She continued, "Have you taken your morning break yet?" He said, "No, I haven't." She replied, "Then you must take one. It's Union policy." He said, "Okay," and followed her to music therapy.

> Mr. Conley had been a construction worker all of his adult life. He busied himself around the facility by attempting to fix things. While he was working, he was completely caught up in his work and was committed to doing a good job.

Music Intervention to Avoid Catastrophic Behavior

Tolerance for sensory stimulation depends in part on whether stimulation occurs at random or whether it has some order. All people have a need for organization and order in their lives (Gaston, 1968), but physically frail, confused, or disoriented people cannot impose order on their own environments. Therefore, they suffer distress when disturbing events occur around them, especially if the events are accompanied by cacophonous sounds. They respond to the noise, clatter, and chaos in the only way they can—with problem behavior.

The results of several studies have indicated that music is an effective intervention for reducing and potentially delaying problem behavior among older adults (Forbes, Peacock, & Morgan, 2005; Gotell, Brown, & Ekman, 2002; Koger, Chapin, & Brotons, 1999). One intervention for problem behavior is to provide periods of time (20–30 minutes each) throughout the day when emotional stress can be diffused. Periods of quiet, except for selected background music, can provide relief from the noise and activity of daily life, which can lead to agitated, emotional behaviors. During these 20- to 30-minute long periods, televisions are turned off, all appliances and other machinery are quieted, lights are turned down low, and agitated people are removed from the area. Music is used to provide organization and order, which contributes to a person's ability to be comfortable during the quiet period. The music must be produced on good-quality sound equipment to encourage interest and commitment to it and to attract attention.

It is also best to use the music that is preferred by the older adults for whom it is intended. However, this preference is difficult to assess in long-term care facilities, where the ages of residents can range from approximately 55 to 100 years and older. In addition, preference differs according to the background and experience of the individual. However, some consistency in types of preferred music can generally be determined. Certain music can be used repetitively until a person develops a familiarity and then a preference for it. Development of the preference takes time and some people may respond slowly at first. Once the music becomes associated with quiet time, comfort, and relaxation, people are drawn to it.

The nursing staff of a residential care unit for people with severe dementia successfully used music to structure quiet time with 28 residents who had difficult-to-manage behaviors. The nurses observed that acting out, wandering, combative behaviors, and emotional outbursts seemed to occur more frequently at certain times of the day, such as near mid-morning bathing and toileting, lunch, just before the afternoon shift change, and when caregivers were unavailable. After consulting with a music therapist, the nurses implemented quiet time with music before these time periods and continued to use it for as long as the behaviors occurred. The nurses turned the lights down low, drew the blinds, and played the music in free field while they encouraged residents to sit down in recliners and rest. At first, only two or three residents remained seated in the room for the duration of the music. However, over a period of several weeks more residents participated in quiet time because they observed other residents participating and imitated them, or because caregivers helped them to participate by sitting with them and holding their hand. Once the pattern was established, residents came into the day room to sit quietly each time the lights were dimmed and the music was played.

Although no research data were gathered, the nurses reported that the residents exhibited fewer emotional outbursts, fewer verbally and physically combative behaviors, and fewer confrontations during the peak times of day when these behaviors had occurred. The nurses have continued to use quiet time and report that their work is easier and staff–resident interactions are more positive when the residents are more relaxed and less emotionally reactive. Particular sedative or stimulative qualities of the music do not seem to affect the quieting responses, but the structure and familiarity provided by the music along with the dimmed light in a quiet environment establish a context for relaxation and calm.

Another intervention for catastrophic behavior is to remove the stimulus (e.g., a caregiver's activity, another person) that triggered it. Sometimes distraction is effective in avoiding outbursts, but distraction is usually not successful once the catastrophic behavior begins to escalate, and it is usually not possible once the behavior becomes full-blown. When behavior reaches a dangerous level, it is possible to introduce a structured intervention that involves singing or speaking in a slow, low-pitched, quiet voice in view of the person, but out of striking range. It is important to sing the most familiar and preferred music of the individual. Spoken commentary can include empathic statements, discussion about the situation, or other remarks that seem appropriate. As the person calms down, the caregiver may want to hold the individual by placing an arm around the shoulders, making sure to stand or sit where the care recipient can readily see his or her face. Recorded music can be used, but accessing the equipment is often awkward and impractical.

This approach is appropriate when the individual's reaction has been triggered by a minor event in the environment (e.g., another person accidentally bumping a shoulder as he or she walks by, someone sitting in the person's favorite chair, someone striking out in confusion). It is not intended for someone who has a strong emotional reaction to an incident (e.g., learning that a loved one has died, being told that placement in the residential care facility is permanent). Events that have strong emotional content require approaches other than that outlined here.

CONCLUSION

Music seems to calm people who have difficult-to-manage behaviors. Staff in residential care facilities often comment that they wait to perform procedures with these individuals until after the music therapist has conducted a session with them. They also comment that these residents seem more coherent after music therapy and can be more easily managed during procedures such as taking their temperature and blood pressure, administering medication, and providing a snack or beverage. The effects of music on the activities and procedures that follow a music therapy session have not been adequately studied. However, there may be some benefit in using music interventions in caregiving regimens (e.g., to structure the environment so as to avoid harmful responses to it and to calm the care recipient should such responses occur).

With or without music, difficult-to-manage behaviors are problematic for both caregivers and care recipients. Both caregivers and care recipients react to the changes associated with aging and with certain progressive conditions or diseases. As these changes take place over time, the approaches that once met care needs become obsolete. Caregivers may respond to the results of this transition with frustration, which may be exacerbated by their fear and panic; care recipients may respond to the results of this transition with resistance or withdrawal.

Relief for both caregivers and care recipients will likely arise from adaptations of the environment and the approaches to care used to meet the challenges of changing care needs. Several principles may help to guide these adaptations:

- Caregivers must be careful to conserve energy.
- Caregivers must set goals for themselves and for their care recipients that are feasible.
- Caregivers must provide as much external structure and predictability as possible, and music may contribute to these qualities.
- Caregivers can observe the responses of their care recipients to determine what factors lead to harmful reactions and what factors result in cooperative behaviors.
- Caregivers can note the times of day when catastrophic behaviors are likely to occur and head them off using positive experiences such as participating in music.
- Caregivers can schedule quiet times with music when harmful reactions are likely to occur.
- Caregivers can become discouraged, frustrated, and hurt when they must cope constantly with difficult situations; it is acceptable for them to ask for help and to not be able to do everything for everyone all the time.

REFERENCES

Aldridge, D. (2007). Dining rituals and music. *Music Therapy Today*, 8(1), 26–38. Retrieved August 1, 2007, from http://musictherapyworld.net

American Psychiatric Association. (2000). *Diagnostic and statistical manual of mental disorders* (4th ed.) Washington, DC: Author.

Clark, M. E., Lipe, A. W., & Bilbrey, M. (1998). Use of music to decrease aggressive behaviors in people with dementia. *Journal of Gerontological Nursing*, 24(7), 10–17.

Cohen-Mansfield, J. (1986). Agitated behaviors in the elderly. II: Preliminary results in the cognitively deteriorated. *Journal of the American Geriatric Society*, 34(10), 722–727.

Dossey, L. (1993). *Healing words: The power of prayer and the practice of medicine*. New York: HarperCollins.

Ebberts, A. G. (1994). *The effectiveness of three types of music therapy interventions with persons diagnosed with probable dementia of the Alzheimer's type who display agitated behaviors*. Unpublished master's thesis, University of Kansas, Lawrence.

Feil, N., & De Klerk-Rubin, V.(2002). *The validation breakthrough: Simple techniques for communicating with people with "Alzheimer's-type dementia"* (2nd ed.). Baltimore: Health Professions Press.

Fitzgerald-Cloutier, M. L. (1993). The use of music therapy to decrease wandering: An alternative to restraints. *Music Therapy Perspectives*, 11(1), 32–36.

Forbes, D. A., Peacock, S., & Morgan, D. (2005). Nonpharmacological management of agitated behaviours associated with dementia. *Geriatrics and Aging*, 8(4), 26–30.

Galasko, D., Schmidt, F., Thomas, R., Jin, S., Bennett, D., & Ferris,S. (2005). Detailed assessment of activities of daily living in moderate to severe Alzheimer's disease. *Journal of the International Neuropsychological Society*, 11(4), 446–453.

Gaston, E. T. (1968). Man and music. In E. T. Gaston (Ed.), *Music in therapy* (pp. 7–29). New York: Macmillan.

Gotell, E., Brown, S., & Ekman, S. L. (2002). Caregiver singing and background music in dementia care. *Western Journal of Nursing Research*, 24(2), 195–216.

Hanser, S. (1990). A music therapy strategy for depressed older adults in the community. *Journal of Applied Gerontology*, 9(3), 283–298.

Isselbacher, K., Braunwald, E., Wilson, J., Martin, J., Fauci, A., & Kasper, D. (Eds.). (1994). *Harrison's principles of internal medicine* (13th ed.). New York: McGraw-Hill.

Kasper, D. L., Braunwald, E., Fauci, A., Hauser, S., Longo, D., & Jameson, J. L. (2004). *Harrison's principles of internal medicine* (16th ed.). Columbus: McGraw-Hill Professional.

Koger, S. M., Chapin, K., & Brotons, M. (1999). Is music therapy an effective intervention for dementia? A meta-analytic review of literature. *The Journal of Music Therapy*, 36(1), 2–15.

Lucero, M. (1995). *Creative interventions with Alzheimer's patients.* Workshop sponsored by ManorCare, the Topeka Chapter of the Alzheimer's Association, and Stormont-Vail Regional Medical Center, Topeka, KS.

Mace, N., & Rabins, P. (1991). *The 36-hour day: A family guide to caring for persons with Alzheimer's disease, related dementing illness and memory loss in later life* (Rev. ed.). Baltimore: The Johns Hopkins University Press.

Mathey, M. F., Vanneste, V. G., de Graaf, C., de Groot, L. C., & van Staveren, W. A. (2001). Health effect of improved meal ambiance in a Dutch nursing home: A 1 year intervention study. *Preventative Medicine*, 32(5), 416–423.

Ropper, A. H., & Brown, R. H. (2005). *Adams and Victor's principles of neurology* (8th ed.). Columbus: McGraw-Hill Professional.

Sadock, B. J., & V. A. Sadock. (2004). *Kaplan & Sadock's comprehensive textbook of psychiatry* (7th ed.). Baltimore: Lippincott Williams & Wilkins.

Selye, H. (1956). *The stress of life.* New York: McGraw-Hill.

Spira, A. P., & Edelstein, B. A. (2006). Behavioral interventions for agitation in older adults with dementia: An evaluative review. *International Psychogeriatrics*, 18(2), 195–225.

Summer, L. (1990). *Guided imagery and music in the institutional setting.* St. Louis, MO: MMB Music.

Thaut, M. (2002). Neuropsychological processes in music perception and their relevance in music therapy. In M. H. Thaut & R. G. Unkefer (Eds.), *Music therapy in the treatment of adults with mental disorders: Theoretical bases and clinical interventions* (pp. 2–32). St. Louis, MO: MMB Music.

Twedell, D., & O'Neil, M. (2007). Depression in the elderly. *The Journal of Continuing Education in Nursing*, 38(1), 14–15.

Chapter 5

$\mathscr{S}$tress and Pain Management through Music

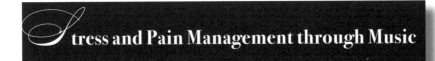

Stress and Pain Management through Music

Whether it is triggered by a situation or an event, stress is perceived by the individual who experiences it as a disturbance of equilibrium. The natural reaction to stress is the "fight or flight" response, which was described by Selye (1956) as a state of arousal that progresses through the following three stages: (1) an alarm reaction in response to the immediate demands of the stressor, (2) either resistance or adaptation to the demands of the stressor, and (3) the depletion of energy or complete exhaustion that comes from continued exposure to the stressor. The physiological changes that accompany stress include increased heart rate, elevated blood pressure, increased respiration rate, decreased skin temperature, increased sweating, decreased gastrointestinal activity, increased or decreased pupil size, and increased muscle tone. When the fight or flight response is suppressed and does not relieve the stress and the influences of the stressors are not disrupted, individuals are held in a constant state of arousal, which leads eventually to impaired physical health and even serious illness, such as heart attack or stroke (Benson, 1992). In addition, stress can lead to the suppression of immunological systems of the body, which increases susceptibility to disease (Blonna, 2006; Bloom, Lazerson, & Nelson, 2005). Several research studies show the potential for the positive influences of music on immunological systems (Bartlett, Kaufman, & Smeltekop, 1993; Hirokawa & Ohira, 2003; Hucklebridge, Lambert, Clow, Awarburton, Evans, & Sherwood, 2000; Miller, 1992; Rider, Achterberg, Lawlis, Goven, Toledo, & Butler, 1990; Tsao, Gordon, Maranto, Lerman, & Murasko, 1991), but further work is needed to determine explicit relationships.

Individuals' abilities to cope with stress depend on past experiences and their coping mechanisms. In addition, the perception of the stressor, its intensity, and the time at which it occurs can all influence how individuals cope. A series of stressors can result in a pyramid effect (Neupert, Almeida, & Charles, 2007; Schober & Affara, 2006), in which stress multiplies as stressors are added one on top of the other. Normal age-related changes also influence how people deal with stressors, and the ability to cope may be altered by sleep deprivation, medications, physical pain, or other factors (Schober & Affara, 2006). Access to family or peer support can also influence any attempts to manage stress. Consequently, the following three areas interact when individuals respond to stressors: (1) the perceptions people have of the stressor and its interpretation in the context of life events, (2) the time of occurrence in relation to other demands, and (3) the access to personal and social resources (Schober & Affara, 2006).

Although stress is harmful, it is also necessary for health and well-being and leads to adjustments in life and personal development (Minois, 2000; Schober & Affara, 2006). Coping with stress, therefore, is a necessary part of life that can lead to satisfaction once appropriate adaptations are made.

Whether stress culminates in satisfactory resolution or in further disequilibrium and anxiety, it is possible to manage the physiological reactions to it by enhancing coping strategies using relaxation and music. Thus, the harmful effects of stress on physical health can be avoided, or at least diminished.

Relaxation can be defined as a state of relative freedom from both anxiety and muscular tension (Benson & Klipper, 2000). In general, relaxation involves physiological responses and is characterized by decreases in heart rate, respiration, oxygen intake, muscle tension, and blood pressure and by increases in alpha brain waves (Benson & Klipper, 2000).

MUSIC AND RELAXATION TECHNIQUES

Music evokes relaxation responses by providing a rhythmic structure for breathing and release of muscle tension, a soothing environment, associations with physical comfort, relief from anxiety through predictability, and a means of implementing some control. Music can be incorporated readily into traditional relaxation approaches, including progressive muscle relaxation (Jacobson, 1938; Robb, 2000), meditative relaxation (Schultz & Luthe, 1969), jaw drop technique (McCaffery & Pasero, 1999), and guided imagery (Bruscia & Grocke, 2002; Leuner, 1978).

It should be noted that relaxation for people in pain is not intended as a substitute for medical intervention. Although relaxation techniques may not relieve pain, they can provide individuals with some control while they offer the opportunity to manage the muscle tension and anxiety that exacerbate pain (Snyder, 1992). Relaxation approaches may not be appropriate for all people, particularly if they show no particular interest in learning how to relax or their orientation to reality is poor. Imagery or meditation should never be used with people who have hallucinations, delusions, or other disturbances in their thought processes.

Progressive Muscle Relaxation

Progressive muscle relaxation, developed by Edmund Jacobson (1938), involves tensing and then relaxing muscle groups. This approach requires physical effort for which some people may not have the energy. Some individuals may find that the physical tension causes even more pain, particularly if they have bone or joint disease. For other people who have little to no experience with any relaxation approach, the tension and relaxation of specific muscle groups may provide some immediate results. They may quickly feel the difference between muscles that are rigidly tense and those that have been relaxed. For other people who may experience disturbed thought processes or other forms of reality disorientation, progressive muscle relaxation can potentially offer a structured approach that has less risk of disturbance than does imagery or meditation. Nevertheless, progressive muscle relaxation must be used with caution in people with poor reality orientation because the technique may trigger hallucinations and/or delusions through its focus on certain muscle groups.

The progressive muscle relaxation process enables individuals to get in touch with their bodies and to begin learning how the body feels when it is tense and when it is somewhat more relaxed. To perform progressive muscle relaxation, individuals should have a quiet, calm environment with subdued lighting and should schedule adequate time. For people who experience distortions in reality, however, the lighting must remain bright enough in order to see clearly what and who is in the room. Even then, this approach may be contraindicated for these individuals. Yet, for most people, music can facilitate the effects of the progressive muscle relaxation technique. This music must have a calming effect, which depends on individual experiences, tastes, and preferences. Therefore, the music that is most suitable for relaxation must be selected by each individual. Once the most suitable music has been identified, the individual associates the consistent use of this music with comfort and the release of tension. Consequently, this music facilitates the relaxation response and amplifies the response through the implementation of the technique. The music may also be continued immediately following the technique to maintain restful comfort for as long as desired.

Initially, a coach may be needed to assist individuals in using the progressive muscle relaxation exercises. The coach either may provide instructions during each session or may make an audio recording of the instructions to be played any time relaxation is needed. After the exercises are learned, it may be possible for individuals to perform them without verbal instruction. Scripts that can be used in the exercises are included in Appendix A. These scripts may be used as written or changed to accommodate the special needs and experiences of particular individuals.

Meditative Relaxation

Meditative relaxation can be either autogenic (from sources within the individual) or structured (through instructions). Autogenic training in meditation began with Schultz and Luthe (1969), who used relaxation and induced images as an approach to psychotherapy. Generally, individuals were left to form their own images and ideas, which could then be incorporated in therapy sessions. Although relaxation was a component of this approach, it was not the focus.

Since the 1950s, self-initiated approaches to relaxation have included meditation, visualization, or images that bring comfort and relief. With this form of relaxation, there is no physical contraction (tightening) of muscle groups. Meditative relaxation begins with a focus on breathing. With each exhaled breath, individuals should think about releasing muscle tension in various body parts. In addition, individuals should imagine a place where they feel safe, secure, and healthy. The technique is enhanced by music, particularly music with which individuals have previously experienced comfort and therefore have associated relief. The music must be compatible with the pattern of breathing; that is, the rhythm of the music must match the pace of the inhalations and exhalations. This rhythmic structure promotes individual attention to stimuli that block pain perception and provides a format for participation. The end of the music indicates the end of the relaxation experience.

Meditative relaxation can be used by individuals whenever they wish. They can use audio-recorded suggestions or cues that remind them to breathe deeply and to remember a place where they felt calm and peaceful. Often, this place differs from individual to individual. For some people, it may be the porch swing at their childhood home, the tree they used to sit in as a youth, their grandmother's rocking chair with the lace arm covers, or their favorite automobile. For other people, it may be a riverbank from which they fished, a hill on which they lay looking at clouds, a favorite park, or the arms of their higher power or God.

Meditative material involves the senses, which are enhanced by music. (See Appendix B for instructions and script suggestions.) Mrs. Sparks, a woman who had not been able to walk for some time and who had severe pain, used meditative relaxation effectively. Initially, she used an audio recording of a script made for her by a music therapist that included her particular comfort experiences and her preferred calming music. After a series of sessions, Mrs. Sparks began to explore doing meditative relaxation with music but without the recorded instructions. She found that the images evoked were stronger and even more involved with sensory experiences than they were with the recorded instructions. In addition, when she saw a particularly pleasant image, she could maintain it for some time to derive even more relaxation and enjoyment from it. Mrs. Sparks explained some of her images to the music therapist:

> I pictured myself on a beach. I don't know where it was, but I was standing in the cold, wet sand. I was barefoot and I could feel it squish up between my toes as I walked along the edge of the water. I felt the coldness, the dampness, an experience I have not been able to enjoy for many years. I also remember the wind in my face blowing my long hair back behind me. The wind was rather cool and damp. As I turned my head, my hair swirled around until I could not see. The wind blew my long, flowing dress of pink chiffon so that it billowed up around my shoulders. With lulls in the wind, I could feel it float down to wrap against my ankles, and when the gusts came, it filled with air like some large, pink cloud.

The woman continued to use her music and the meditative relaxation technique to enhance these visualizations and to experience others. She said that the only time she could enjoy the experience of moving freely was when she used the music and the relaxation technique. She also reported that she enjoyed the personal control over physical discomfort that the technique provided.

Although meditative relaxation is not appropriate for all people, it has excellent potential for the relief of pain or anxiety. It should never be used with people who have poor concepts of reality, and it may be beyond the grasp of people who do not have an interest in or motivation for trying it.

Jaw Drop Technique

The jaw drop technique (see Appendix D) is simple and requires little training to learn to use it well. This approach is particularly effective in mediating moderate to severe pain in older adults, especially if it is practiced before pain is felt (McCaffery & Pasero, 1999). Because the technique involves relaxing the tongue, it must be used only when the head is somewhat elevated to avoid blockage of the airway. In the jaw drop technique, relaxation spreads from the face, jaw, and tongue to the rest of the body. The effects of this technique may be enhanced using music selected to fit individual breathing rhythms and preferences for style and type of music. The music that is associated with comfort is the music that is most likely to facilitate relief during the jaw drop exercise. Thus, music must be individually selected for people who would like to use music accompaniment with this technique.

Guided Imagery

Imagery techniques have been found to be effective in the management of chronic pain (Snyder, 1992). Theoretically, this effectiveness results from enhanced endorphin (substance in the brain that mediates pain) secretion and disrupted processing of pain information in the brain (Korn, 1983). People who find that thoughts or images can alter their perceptions of pain may also find that these perceptual alterations can be enhanced by listening to appropriate music.

Optimal relief through the use of imagery is achieved with experience and practice. Guided imagery (images that are evoked through verbal suggestion) may speed the process, but relief may be hampered if the material is not particularly significant to the individual who attempts to use it. Relief is greatest when people integrate their own experiences and associations into the images and form personal attachments to them than when they integrate other people's experiences and associations. External suggestions have limited personal value and may even evoke unpleasant thoughts or fears. With the possibility of such strong reactions, it is essential to consider each person's belief system and past experiences before selecting guided imagery as a relaxation approach for pain remediation. Some people who hold fundamentalist religious beliefs consider any external suggestion of pictures, thoughts, or images as evil. Consequently, guided imagery can evoke fear, anxiety, and emotional reactivity in some persons by merely mentioning it as a pain management technique. It is recommended that individuals use their own ideas and thoughts without employing suggestions from others, and that any commercially produced audio recordings that claim to provide guided imagery appropriate to pain management be examined with caution. (See Appendix C for visualization with relaxation instructions and script suggestions.)

The inherent danger in using external guides for images is their power to evoke memories or experiences that are potentially harmful. During these experiences, stress can increase as can the severity of pain. The power of images is particularly strong when music is used because music enhances the effects of the technique used and triggers thoughts and memories associated with it, whether or not they are pleasant or desirable. The following is an example of harmful guided imagery, which was used by Mrs. Lewis, an anesthetist. Before administering anesthesia, Mrs. Lewis used one image for all patients, regardless of personal preference or background.

> I am about to give you something to relax you through the intravenous port in your arm. I would like for you to picture yourself on the shore of a very large lake or on the beach at the ocean. As I introduce the drug, you will begin to feel cold. I want you to imagine yourself walking into the water. Feel it

becoming colder and darker as you walk deeper and deeper into it. Feel the cold water come up over your head as you are submerged completely in the cold darkness.

Although it is unlikely, this image may have been pleasant for some patients. However, many patients felt fear and anxiety. Patients who were afraid of deep water, who feared drowning, and who generally did not enjoy the sensation of the cold or darkness most likely had negative associations with Mrs. Lewis' script.

Another potentially harmful script was used with Mrs. Silbert, who was receiving palliative pain management in a hospice. She had begun to experience severe discomfort and was hospitalized suddenly. She was agitated about leaving her home without making adequate preparations. Mrs. Silbert had always believed that she would have time to clean and straighten her house before she had to leave it. Ms. Horkey, a young music therapy student who had training in relaxation and pain management techniques, talked with her about using deep breathing and imagery to alleviate her discomfort. Mrs. Silbert agreed to try the approach. After selecting music that had a calming effect and after coaching Mrs. Silbert in rhythmic breathing, Ms. Horkey began reciting the following commonly used script:

> Picture yourself in a beautiful, cool meadow. It is high in the mountains. The air is clean and fresh and it feels cool as it blows against your skin. There are wildflowers everywhere, and they are all colors of the rainbow.

Mrs. Silbert interrupted Ms. Horkey, saying frantically, "Get me out of here! I can't stand being in this meadow! All I can think about is lying beneath the sod in my grave. I can't breathe with the dirt on my face. Help me! Stop!" Ms. Horkey immediately terminated the guided imagery and asked Mrs. Silbert if there was something she would rather think about as they listened to music. Mrs. Silbert related her disappointment about leaving her house in "such an uproar," and said that she would really like to clean her kitchen cupboards.

The student listened to Mrs. Silbert as she described each cupboard, its location in the kitchen, and the contents of each shelf. Ms. Horkey took notes for items Mrs. Silbert wanted to give to family and for the actual cleaning tasks Mrs. Silbert knew family members would have to do after her passing. Ms. Horkey and Mrs. Silbert went through all the items in all the cabinets, designating contents to Mrs. Silbert's satisfaction. As they completed these tasks, they listened to music, including "The Irish Washer Woman," one of Mrs. Silbert's favorite songs. Mrs. Silbert continued her kitchen work over a series of sessions. Occasionally, she would clap her hands in time to the music and talk about some of the memories she associated with it. Once she finished the kitchen, she moved on to the closets, and then to the drawers. Eventually, she imagined the entire house cleaned, put in order, and ready for her to leave it.

Ms. Horkey was able to adapt her approach to the needs and desires of a woman discomforted not only by her physical pain but also by her anxiety about her sudden hospitalization. This adaptation was an appropriate use of the guided imagery technique in that the guide interacted with the woman and did not push her or direct the associations and images that surfaced.

Guided Imagery and Music (GIM)

Guided Imagery and Music (GIM) is a technique that powerfully influences emotional responses and therefore has the potential for either beneficial or harmful effects. Whether positive or negative, the effect of Guided Imagery and Music lies in the competence of the guide, and professional training is essential. The Bonny Foundation (among other organizations) has designed programs to train individuals in three levels of Guided Imagery and Music. Successful completion of each level provides the background and skill necessary to use these clinical applications in a specific context.

MUSIC IN MANAGING PAIN AND ANXIETY

Pain is classified into two major categories: acute and chronic (McCaffery & Pasero, 1999). *Acute pain* refers to pain that subsides as healing occurs and thus has a predictable end. Acute pain generally lasts no longer than 6 months, may have a slow or sudden onset, and can range in intensity from mild to severe (e.g., pain associated with amputation, surgery, bone fractures, infections). *Chronic pain* generally lasts 6 months or longer and is characterized by recurrent acute pain that occurs over a prolonged time period or a lifetime (e.g., migraine headaches that occur once or twice a week for months or years); ongoing time-limited pain (e.g., pain associated with cancer or burns); and chronic benign (nonmalignant) pain that is not life-threatening, does not respond to pain relief methods, and may continue over a lifetime (e.g., pain associated with vascular disease, rheumatoid arthritis, osteoporosis).

The relief of pain is a priority for people who experience acute or chronic pain. This pain or discomfort can be either localized (in one specific area) or generalized (throughout the body). It may or may not have a clear etiology (cause), but it is nonetheless real to the person who experiences it. Whatever the source, pain is exacerbated by muscle tension, anxiety, and other types of emotional distress (McCaffery & Pasero, 1999). Effective management of pain must incorporate whatever interventions bring relief when used either alone or in combination. At the heart of this relief is the control of anxiety and emotional distress.

The most commonly accepted intervention for pain is the administration of pharmacological agents, but the effects of these agents may be limited because of individualized experiences of pain or discomfort. Individuals may have differences in pain thresholds, slower metabolic processing in older people as compared to younger people, differences in the effects of some pharmacological agents from person to person, and varying side effects, which may include drowsiness or loss of consciousness. Older people can respond negatively to medication because the prolonged drug activity that is typical in older adults can lead to accumulation (Malseed, Goldstein, & Balkon, 1995); the alterations in renal and hepatic functioning can result in toxicity (Zhan et al., 2001); and the decreased cardiac output, decreased hepatic activity, altered gastrointestinal functioning, decreased body weight, fat displacement of muscle, and lowered plasma albumin levels can influence the effects of the medication (Zhan et al., 2001). Administration of any pain medication can cause additional medical problems if harmful side effects occur, particularly if the medication interacts nontherapeutically with other drugs the person is taking.

Ameliorating pain and discomfort is the primary goal for the medical staff that works with people in pain, and pharmacological interventions alone may be inadequate (McCaffery & Pasero, 1999; Schober & Affara, 2006). There are some indications that the pharmacological effects of analgesics and narcotics may be enhanced by relaxation, distraction, and other stimuli (McCaffery & Pasero, 1999; Schober & Affara, 2006). These stimuli are particularly important when the most effective medication or combination of medications has not been determined, the dosage has become inadequate because a person has developed an increased tolerance to the medication, or the frequency of dose administration does not provide sufficient relief. It is essential that the person's physician be informed when medications are ineffective or insufficient so that appropriate changes can be made; the lag time between such adjustments and their effects may leave people with discomfort, which can be managed only by alternative means. These alternatives can include cutaneous stimulation through the application of hot or cold temperatures, which may be combined with massage; the implementation of relaxation techniques; the use of imagery; the application of music as a distraction (McCaffery & Pasero, 1999); and the use of music as a relaxation and stress management enhancer.

Essential to the effective management of pain is implementing an intervention before a level of discomfort is reached (McCaffery & Pasero, 1999). Timing an intervention appropriately will increase its effectiveness and will avert the ever-increasing intensity of the discomfort and the anxiety that builds with it. Without early intervention, people feel pain longer, and the effectiveness of medication and other approaches are compromised as the discomfort and the tension that accompanies it build. This concept applies in all cases where pain management is an issue, whether it is acute or chronic.

In general, people develop patterns in their experiences of pain so that they come to know when pain will occur and when it will increase. Consequently, people can learn when the implementation of a particular intervention will be most effective. Interventions of particular interest are the uses of music as a distraction and as a relaxation enhancer, both of which can amplify the effects of pharmacological management. These interventions are in no way intended as substitutes for medication; rather, they are intended for use in conjunction with medication to increase or prolong its effects.

Management of physical pain with music has basis in new

research that demonstrates how a small, almond-shaped part of the brain, the amygdala, functions in pain perception. This research demonstrates that a relationship exists between persistent pain and negative emotions such as fear (Neugebauer, 2004) making the amygdala central to sensory and emotional pain processing (Pedersen, Scheel-Krüger, Blackburn-Munro, 2007). Therefore, it is possible that when the perception of fear is diminished through engagement in music, the perception of pain is also diminished. Further research has demonstrated a clinically well-documented relationship between pain and anxiety and the amygdala, though the full function of the amygdala in the interaction of pain and anxiety is still not clear (Ji, Fu, Ruppert, & Neugebauer, 2007).

Research evidence shows that both acute pain and chronic pain are managed by the amygdala (Carrasquillo & Gereau, 2007; Ikeda, Takahashi, Kazuhine, & Kato, 2007; Ji & Negebauer, 2007), though mechanisms employed by the amygdala are different in perceptions of acute, chronic, neuropathic, and inflammatory pain (Neugebauer, 2007) and in the acquisition and retention of fear (Baker & Kim, 2004). Further, Neugebauer (2007) speculates that the amygdala is a pain facilitator that allows pain perception when pain is a primary concern; but, in a life-threatening situation, whether it is real or perceived, the amygdala suppresses pain perception as attention is directed toward "fight or flight" in an effort to guarantee survival.

In a very simple explanation, this body of research demonstrates that the amygdala, located deep inside the brain, is activated when it receives signals that indicate pain and the emotions that are associated with it, for example, fear, anxiety, and depression. When the amygdala is stimulated by these signals, it sends messages on to upper parts of the brain that recognize the messages. If the amygdala is kept from reacting as strongly to the initial signals, for instance, if it is quieted by music, it sends far weaker pain and pain-associated emotional messages to the upper parts of the brain. As a result, a person's pain sensations are greatly reduced and he or she feels more comfortable.

The influence of music to stimulate the brain to register strongly pleasant emotional responses is well-known (Blood & Zatorre, 2001). More recent brain mapping while listening to music, however, has indicated differences in responses to pleasant and un-pleasant music. This research demonstrates that unpleasant music activates the amygdala, hippocampus, parahippocampal gyrus, and temporal poles in an unpleasant emotional response. Pleasant music, however, activates other brain structures, including the inferior fron-tal gyrus, the anterior superior insula, the ventral striatum, Heschi's gyrus, and the Rolandic operculum, resulting in pleasant emotional responses (Koelsch, Fritz, Cramon, Müller, & Frederici, 2006). It is important to recognize that pleasant and unpleasant music each stim-ulate the brain in different ways and both are of sufficient strength for either a positive or a negative emotional perception. Therefore, the use of music through listening, or other forms of active music participation, must be evaluated for levels of pleasant or unpleasant emotional responses for individual participants. It would seem that as pleasant music stimulates positive emotional responses, individuals' perceptions of fear, anxiety, and pain may decrease. This gives pain-managing drugs time to work and actually may even help them work. Music can be used to alter the perception of pain in several ways, in-cluding, but not limited to, providing structure; diversion from bore-dom; stimulation of thoughts, ideas, and memories; and, for some people, a way to interact with other people.

Providing Structure

People who are in pain may find their perceptions of it in-crease as time passes. For many, time seems to stand still. They con-tinue to focus their attention on the slowly moving clock as well as their discomfort, which seems to grow with each passing moment. Involvement in music may provide relief; however, once the pain has mounted, people will likely require assistance to refocus their atten-tion on the music and away from their discomfort. In addition, people who have nothing to do except think about how uncomfortable they are may find that their pain increases as they continue to focus on it. Any diversion from this focus can help people alleviate their discom-fort, at least for a time.

People who have severe discomfort may find listening to music annoying because they cannot engage their attention in order to respond to it adequately. Guided listening may provide sufficient structure for them to respond when they are asked to listen for certain themes, lyrics, or other musical elements. A music therapist may conduct guided listening after carefully assessing a person's musical preferences. Using preferred musical selections, the introduction to listening and subsequent engagement in the music may occur as follows:

> The music therapist says, "I have with me (*title of song, sonata, opera, other*). I understand it is some of your favorite music. I am going to play a bit of this for you and I want you to raise your hand when you hear (*instrumentation, song lyric, other*)." The music therapist plays the example. Once the individual responds, the therapist draws attention to other specific elements of the music and indicates how the person may respond, either verbally or nonverbally. Timing is essential and minimal explanation is provided to allow spontaneous engagement. As participation continues, the music therapist may shift to other forms of involvement (e.g., listening for certain phrases, timbres, concepts). The therapist may find it necessary to provide some examples, such as "I really like the way (*name of the performer*) sings this phrase. I want you to hear it." The therapist plays the phrase. "What do you think? Did you like it? What about it particularly impressed you? How about hearing more?" The music therapist either continues with the selection or shifts to a selection that may be more effective in capturing the individual's attention.

If people cannot participate in the guided listening because their discomfort is too advanced, live singing may distract individuals from their focus on pain. A music therapist can implement this approach at bedside, either standing or sitting close to the individual to facilitate eye contact. The music therapist can also instruct the caregiver(s) to utilize this technique. For the best outcome, songs that are preferred by the person should be used. Singing can begin after a simple introduction, such as "I'm going to sing to you now," accompanied by the request, "Can you look at me?" Singing is implemented whether or not individuals open their eyes, and generally eye contact is not made until after some time. Songs must continue long enough to allow response to them, and it is important that portions of songs that are the most familiar are sung (e.g., the first verse and the chorus, or only the chorus). Accompaniment is not required; in fact, an accompaniment may be disturbing because its sound is perhaps too harsh to evoke desirable responses. However, accompaniment may benefit some people, adding to the distraction, which therefore may yield relief. The potential for positive responses using accompaniment can be explored. Individuals' reactions to the instruments must be observed closely to determine which sound stimuli are the most soothing.

As the bedside singing continues and individuals make eye contact, additional forms of participation may serve as distractions. Individuals may be asked to sing along, to move to the music (e.g., tap a finger, wiggle a toe, wave a hand, nod the head), or to play the finger cymbals, Omnichord, or some other instrument that requires little effort apart from active engagement through a structured, rhythmic response. This participation requires individuals to focus on their musical productivity from moment to moment rather than on their pain. Therefore, they may not perceive as much discomfort. When pain subsides, guided listening may be used to maintain individuals' comfort levels and to induce relaxation, rest, or even sleep.

Providing a Diversion from Boredom

As people begin to learn to focus on listening to certain elements of their music, they may no longer need a coach or guide. They may need to periodically consult with a coach to determine which approach best facilitates active listening, and they may also explore approaches on their own. When people are actively listening and not watching the clock, they move through time as they move through the music. They do not focus on their discomfort out of lack of anything to do. It must be noted, however, that this approach is effective only as long as they are actively engaged. Attention cannot be maintained indefinitely and will eventually wane. Some people are able to listen actively for several hours, but other people are able to maintain attention for only 20–30 minutes or less.

No matter what the individual attention span is, intermittent silence can shift the focus to the music whenever it is reintroduced. In addition, changing the selections to different types or styles of music can provide novelty, which can hold attention longer. Periods of silence between periods of active listening throughout the day can help listeners to avoid fatigue and to alter the adaptation process that occurs with any stimulation, including music, over time.

Other ways of using music as distraction from pain, particularly acute pain, include: singing a song or a phrase of a song aloud repeatedly until the pain subsides; singing a song or a phrase and tapping out the rhythm with a finger; and singing a song or a phrase repeatedly mentally until the pain subsides (McCaffery & Pasero, 1999). The general rule is to increase the stimulation as the perception of pain increases; to redirect a person's focus to rhythm, which distracts attention from the pain; and to engage individuals in pain as actively as possible with consideration given to their energy level and their state of mind. McCaffery and Pasero (1999) also recommend stimulating the senses simultaneously to provide the best distraction (e.g., listening to or making music for auditory stimulation while also tapping out rhythm for kinesthetic stimulation; holding or touching something for tactile stimulation; looking at a point on the wall or ceiling or forming a mental visual image for visual stimulation).

The self-initiated singing and tapping out rhythm intervention requires a minimal amount of instruction. This instruction can be conducted as follows:

> A music therapist approaches an individual by calling his or her name and directing his or her attention by saying, "Hello," softly at first and then more loudly until the person effects some type of facial response or movement (e.g., grimace, turn of the head, eye contact). The person is told, "I'm going to sing to you." A familiar song, such as "Home on the Range," or a preferred song, is sung. Again, loudness levels of singing and speaking are adjusted to the person's responsiveness, which is tied to the intensity of the pain, for example, louder with less responsiveness and more pain, and softer with more responsiveness and less pain. The person is further directed to "Sing out loud or in your thoughts with me and tap your finger to the beat." At this point, a familiar chorus of a song is sung repeatedly, and the therapist taps the individual's fingers or hand to the beat while singing. The singing and tap-

ping continue while the person engages in rhythmic tapping and singing, if desired. The person is again encouraged to sing with the therapist and to tap out the rhythm. This verbal cue is provided intermittently until finger tapping begins and is continued. Singing continues until the individual indicates verbally that the pain has subsided. Other indications of decreased pain will also be evident, such as relaxed hands and feet, lowered shoulders, slowed breathing, neutral facial expressions, and perhaps sleep. Although sleep (when not drug-induced and occurring in conjunction with physical relaxation) does not always indicate the relief of pain, it is likely an outcome of pain relief.

Once the individual is taught how to focus on and tap out the rhythm of the music, directions can be given in self-initiating the mental or vocal singing with rhythmic tapping anytime the person feels discomfort and in increasing the tempo if the pain continues. In addition, the person may be directed to tap fingers on both hands, nod his or her head, or move any body part rhythmically as he or she sings faster. As the pain abates, the person may slow the singing and decrease the tapping. When a person cannot manage self-initiation, he or she can be directed to do so by family or by anyone in attendance.

Providing Stimulation of Thoughts, Ideas, and Memories

Another self-initiated distraction using music is to select music from past life experiences that are generally positive and affirming (e.g., the music couples danced to while dating, the music listened to at home when the family was together, the songs sung to children and grandchildren as they grew and matured). Individuals can begin the music, recline, close their eyes, and remember the details associated with the music (e.g., the people, faces, activities, events, sounds, smells, physical sensations, temperature). This approach can be used for 1 hour or more to structure time and to stimulate thoughts that are not related to pain and pain sensations.

These thoughts and memories either can be verbalized as they occur with the music or can be visualized mentally for the moment. If they are verbalized, a caregiver or another person can facilitate reminiscence by asking for details. Audio or video recordings made of verbal descriptions of memories can preserve them so they can be used again to stimulate reminiscence or played to distract a person from severe physical discomfort. In the example that follows, a woman used music to revive memories and relieve discomfort. She referred to her pain as "time to go dancing." The more she listened to the music, the more effective it became as a source of comfort and even pleasure.

> As a diversion from her pain, Mrs. Garinther, a widow with severe arthritis, listened to dance music that was popular when she was young. She said that there were several tunes that particularly reminded her of her husband and that was the music she used as a diversion. When she heard the music, she said that she felt as if he was with her. She said she could almost feel his touch and smell his sweet breath. Mrs. Garinther described going dancing with her husband when they were young. They had a shiny black 1949 Mercury that was his pride and joy. It had fender skirts and curb feelers and was so nice to ride in. When they went dancing, he parked the car far away from the dance hall to avoid dents in the doors from other cars parked next to it. The Mercury had wool seats that were soft to the touch and were never cold in the wintertime. The glow of the dashboard lights at night was a soft yellow, and there was always music on the radio. Often Mr. Garinther sang along, and he loved to serenade her. He sang while he drove, turning his head now and then to catch glimpses of her. His singing and his gestures would become increasingly animated until she smiled. He was always so pleased when he could make her smile. And what a dancer! She could still feel how he held her firmly around her waist and placed his broad, strong hand on her back. They would glide across the floor. It seemed as though her feet never touched the floor as they moved together. Dancing with him almost took her breath away, and it made all her cares and concerns disappear. It was as if no one but them was in the world, as the room blurred past them.

As they danced, she could smell the faint scent of his skin as her cheek touched his. His face was smooth and cool, and in his arms she felt that nothing could ever harm her. He made heaven on earth, and she sensed it most when they danced.

Providing Interaction with Other People

Although memories evoked by music likely distract from pain, sharing these memories may enhance their value by providing opportunities to interact with other people. Sharing these memories can maintain family histories, communicate feelings and thoughts, describe dreams, provide a sense of closeness with cherished people, articulate values, and contribute to family legacies. Some people discover information that would otherwise remain hidden, and other people recall memories that bring them comfort.

Reminiscences that incorporate all stages of life and the music that accompanied them are possible with time and practice, and listening to the music repeatedly can amplify details. Used consistently, reminiscence with music and provision of opportunities to share memories with other people can be valuable sources of diversion, relief, and enhancement of quality of life for people in pain.

MUSIC IN INTENSIVE CARE

Several researchers have examined the positive effects of music in decreasing the anxiety of patients in hospital intensive care units (Voss, Good, Yates, Baun, Thompson, & Hertzog, 2004; White, 1992), increasing their ability to relax (Almerud & Petersson, 2003; Guzzetta, 1989), diverting their attention and decreasing their need for drug therapy (O'Sullivan, 1991; Wilkins & Moore, 2004), and increasing their positive mood (Davis-Rollans & Cunningham, 1987; McDermott & O'Callaghan, 2004) and well-being (McDermott & O'Callaghan, 2004; Updike, 1990). Music in the intensive care unit can be a source of security and familiarity in a frightening environment over which patients have no control. Music can soothingly mask the sounds and activities in the room, provide predictability and calm when surrounded by continuous urgent activity, relieve anxiety and fear, and restore a sense of well-being. Music can also be used by family members and loved ones to relieve their stress during visits by relaxing the patient and relaxing themselves when they are away from the patient. (See Appendices for information on relaxation.)

In general, much of the discomfort for patients in the intensive care unit arises from feeling a sense of powerlessness that they are not able to control or manage their situation, their self-care, or the outcome of their treatment. Powerlessness causes stress via the loss of ability to make decisions and the loss of participation in routine self-care. In addition, feelings of powerlessness and depression are associated with the physical deterioration that occurs despite medical intervention (Urden, Stacy, & Lough, 2005). Large differences exist in the amount of control patients want, and this desire for control seems to diminish with age (Urden et al., 2005). Some people can be overwhelmed by decisions, whereas others want to assume responsibility for them. Therefore, the attribution of control to patients in intensive care units must fit their particular abilities and desires. The option to refuse control must also be offered as a possibility (Rodin, 1986).

Because they feel powerless, patients in intensive care are exposed to a wide range of stressors, including the threat of death and the threat of survival with severe residual problems; experiences of pain; insufficient sleep; boredom; and continual exposure to noise, lights, and the flurry of activity in the care of other patients. Additional stressors come from losses associated with altered family and work roles, deprived privacy, reduced personal dignity, limited or no access to the usual coping mechanisms, compromised abilities to express oneself, and limited or no interaction with loved ones (Urden et al., 2005).

Patients may or may not cope effectively with these stressors in intensive care. Effective coping is predicated on the resources to which they had access before hospitalization and their ability to access them in a time of severe distress. Coping can be defined as the ability of individuals to use both cognitive and behavioral resources to manage specific external and internal demands that either tax or exceed their resources (Aldwin & Werner, 2007). Typically, coping involves using the mechanisms for problem solving and anxiety management that were effective in the past (Urden et al., 2005). If these mechanisms are not adequate in the intensive care situation, specific approaches may be used to provide alternative mechanisms, including preferred music as a diversion, a distraction, and as a relaxation enhancer.

Individuals who cannot provide information concerning their preferred music because of the severity of their medical conditions may still respond to familiar music with alert responses, if not with full consciousness. Conferences with family and loved ones can yield information concerning the patient's preferred music. Loved ones will likely respond eagerly and will provide audio recordings that nurses can use with their patients. With consultation and guidance, families and friends may also assume an active role in organizing and providing musical and relaxation experiences during their visits with their loved one(s). These efforts can provide the structure and focus for visits when conversation is difficult or impossible. In addition, when families and friends provide musical experiences for their loved one(s), they play a meaningful role in the healing process. As a result, they feel needed and purposeful, not helpless. The stress associated with their caregiving role can abate somewhat as they provide constructive assistance and support to the nursing staff. By implementing music programming, loved ones can be integrated with clear purpose into the treatment regimen, and emotional reactions to the circumstance can be more readily managed. Consequently, patients will likely sense the positive, secure environment and will respond favorably to it.

Whether managed by the visiting family or by the nursing staff, the music used must provide comfort and familiarity to the patient. To be effective, the individual who hears it must like it. Furthermore, the individual must adhere to a schedule of intermittent playing to elicit alert responses and to a schedule of continuous playing to enhance or encourage sleep. The sedative and stimulative qualities of the music must also be considered in order to effect desired outcomes.

Music used to encourage relaxation must suit the breathing rhythms and the particular responses of the patient. Family or nursing staff may guide the patient through relaxation exercises and may make an audio recording of the session for use in their absence. The recording may be used whenever the patient wishes and may be particularly comforting because a familiar voice coaches the relaxation exercises over familiar, preferred music. (See Appendices for scripts and exercises.)

MUSIC AND THE TREATMENT OF BURNS

Using music to manage the severe pain of burns is a fairly recent application in pain management. It has proven beneficial in several research studies (Fratianne, Presner, Huston, Super, Yowler, & Standley, 2001; Presner, Yowler, Smith, Steele, & Fratianne, 2001; Whitehead-Pleaux, Baryza, & Sheridan, 2006). Music may be used in the treatment of burns to remediate severe, excruciating pain; distract from the trauma experienced; relieve the sensation of itching; establish comforting human contact; provide predictability and security in an disturbing and disruptive environment; offer inner comfort, peace, and spiritual well-being instead of fear; provide a source of emotional expression; and provide a source for rejoicing and celebration.

The pain associated with severe burns is excruciating and indescribable and subsequently stresses individuals with burn wounds. Although this pain can be somewhat dulled with medication, it mounts with stress and tension and can never be totally eliminated. The pain felt by people with severe burns goes beyond physical discomfort to emotional pain. Some people suffer from post-traumatic stress, with recurrent nightmares and visualizations of their injuries (Powers, Cruse, Daniels, & Stevens, 1994). The burns may be the result of an accident (e.g., they may have set their clothing on fire while burning trash, they may have dropped a boiling tea kettle and splashed scalding water on themselves, they may have fallen asleep with a lit cigarette) or through abuse.

The ability of any patient in intensive care to cope with physical pain, emotional distress, and the circumstances surrounding hospitalization depends on previously developed coping mechanisms. People who have drawn on resources within themselves, such as spiritual beliefs and faith, the ability to divert attention, or any other emotional or physical mechanism, can access their coping abilities. People who do not have this experience will require guidance and coaching to receive relief. Music as a distraction and a diversion may be helpful and relaxation techniques can be effective.

Using Music During Dressing Changes

Dressings of burn wounds must be changed frequently and

the damaged tissue cleaned and cut away. The pain involved is tremendous and seems to be exacerbated by the anxiety, fear, and physical stress and tension people feel in association with the process. A therapeutic technique involving singing as a point of focus has been used effectively by board-certified music therapist Della Clayton Molloy to decrease patients' ratings of pain perception, even when medication dosages were either decreased or eliminated altogether (Clayton, 1995). Clayton Molloy met with patients at least 30 minutes before the dressings were changed. She provided either live or recorded music to redirect their focus. Patients who possessed sufficient cognitive ability to follow her directives were coached in deep, rhythmic breathing and helped to focus on relaxing by releasing the tension in their bodies. (See Appendix B for script suggestions.) Patients who could not follow the coaching directives were provided familiar songs in order to structure their environment, which produced a calming effect. Once relaxed and calmed, patients were left with recorded music playing in order to maintain their level of comfort until the dressing change began.

At the time of the dressing change, Clayton Molloy sang to patients. Holding one or both of their hands against her chest, she sang familiar songs while she tapped out the rhythm of the song on their hands. She changed songs whenever patients indicated with facial expressions or groans their growing discomfort. Clayton Molloy verbally cued patients intermittently to look at her as she sang, and often patients spontaneously sang with her. While she sang and tapped out rhythms and patients focused their attention on her, the dressing changes were completed. Medical staff commented that they were able to finish the procedure in dramatically less time with minimal distress experienced by patients. Patients rated their pain perceptions after the singing lower than before, and all people involved in the procedure sensed relief from the stress associated with the physically painful experience.

Using Music During Debridement

In order to heal, the burned tissue must be debrided, or removed. Debridement encourages the growth of new tissue. The procedure is performed either in surgery or in hydrotherapy, where damaged skin is cut or scrubbed away. (Patients in hydrotherapy are immersed in tubs of water or are sprayed with water while they lie on a gurney.) The procedure is painful and medications are used to dull the pain. Clayton (1995) found music therapy intervention to be viable and efficacious as a distraction from pain. She combined the process of listening to music with deep, rhythmic breathing and either progressive relaxation, meditative relaxation, or visual imagery techniques (see Appendices A, B, and C). Choices of music were made by the patients, and Clayton Molloy coached patients in implementing the choices.

Once patients were relaxed, they were ready to move to the debridement tanks or gurneys. After patients were positioned, Clayton Molloy used whatever distraction technique was found to be the most effective with the individual patients, including having them sing loudly along with her, listening to music played progressively louder as the pain increased, and listening to music up to the point of feeling severe pain, followed by silence as the patient concentrated on an image or a thought. Whatever approach was employed depended upon individual responses and abilities to participate. In some patients, several approaches were used until desired results were achieved.

MUSIC AND MANAGING THE DISCOMFORT AND ANXIETY ASSOCIATED WITH LUNG DISEASE

The two most common diseases of the lung are cancer and chronic obstructive pulmonary disease (COPD), which includes emphysema and chronic bronchitis. Cancer of the lung is the leading cause of cancer deaths in the United States (U.S. Cancer Statistics Working Group, 2007). In 2003, 89,906 men and 68,084 women died from lung cancer. (U.S. Cancer Statistics Working Group, 2007). Chronic obstructive pulmonary disease affected more than 5% of the adult population in 2003. Furthermore, cigarette smoking is attributed to 80% of those diagnosed with this disease (Sin, McAlister, Man, & Anthonisen, 2003).

People with diseases of the lung often have difficulty catching their breath. Breathing can be difficult when they are relaxed, and when they feel stress, either through physical exertion or emotional reaction, the difficulty becomes progressive. The most common complaint of people with respiratory disease is the anxiety caused by shortness of breath related to physical exertion or frequent coughing spells (Gosselink, 2004). These people enter into a cycle of distress where physical exertion required to walk from one room to another in the home leads quickly to breathing distress. Initial difficulties in breathing lead to anxiety. As the anxiety builds, breathing becomes increasingly difficult. As breathing becomes more difficult, anxiety mounts.

Progressive relaxation is effective in relieving distress, which likely occurs when relaxation of the striated muscle (the muscle controlling voluntary function) generalizes to the smooth muscle (the muscle that performs functions not under voluntary control). Subsequently, spasms in the bronchi and the bronchioles are reduced (Gosselink, 2004). Using relaxation to control these spasms reduces anxiety and provides the means to disrupt the cycle of distress. (For scripts, see Appendix A.) People with difficulty in breathing will generally respond best when the progressive relaxation exercises are conducted while they are in a sitting position, as opposed to a reclining position, in order to maximize lung capacity with each breath.

Another approach to relief of breathing distress focuses on slowing the rhythm of breathing and physically relaxing by releasing tension. When music accompanies the rhythmic breathing, the results can be even more satisfying. Although rhythmic breathing is a rather simple concept, the specific physical and emotional conditions of patients make it essential to consult with a qualified health professional in order to determine the appropriate application and adaptation.

Once the specific breathing exercise is determined, the music that will be used to accompany the exercise must be selected to match the desired relaxed breathing rhythm. It must be individually determined. Exploring various musical selections is necessary to make the best choice. This music must be unsyncopated and rhythmically consistent throughout, and other musical elements must also maintain continuity (e.g., no sudden changes in percussiveness, instrumentation, tonality, timbre, tempo).

The music used in rhythmic breathing must also bring emotional comfort to the individual. It is essential that this music evokes feelings of well-being and avoids any strong emotional reactions, whether associated with excitement and pleasure, agitation, sadness, grief, or other strong emotions that can increase stress. Although it may be impossible to avoid all emotional reactions to a piece of music, these emotions must not interfere with the relaxation process. If a selection causes any distraction from the relaxation response, it must be discontinued and another selection found.

For some people, the best music for relaxation of breathing is unfamiliar music with which they have no previous emotional association. For other people, the best music may be the music that has previously relaxed and comforted them. Careful trials with music will reveal which selections are the most successful in remediating anxiety and promoting relaxed breathing. Regular practice of relaxed breathing exercises with music will provide a well-rehearsed approach to managing episodes of respiratory distress when they occur and may help to prevent them. Proper management is contingent upon early implementation. Relaxation exercises with music must be implemented at the first indication of discomfort. When exercises are introduced early enough, anxiety and tension can be diminished and the cycle of distress disrupted. When people successfully manage difficulty in breathing, they gain confidence in their ability to control their reactions to stress, which adds to their sense of comfort and well-being.

Although proper management is contingent upon early intervention, individuals may not always have access to their music at the onset of an episode of distress in breathing (e.g., at a public gathering or outside the home where a compact disc player is not available). At these times, music can be played mentally and breathing exercises implemented, provided the approach is well rehearsed. Individuals should have a plan in place to move to a quiet area if possible. The plan may include a cue to indicate whether the person in distress would like to have company. If the plan includes the accompaniment of another person, it should have nonverbal cues given by the other person to indicate methods of relaxation. The accompanying person must be a source of comfort, not a source of distraction (e.g., the accompanying person attempts to engage the person in distress in a conversation, or becomes frightened or alarmed by the distress). This person must remain calm, gently guide the person in distress to a quiet place, and safeguard the individual's privacy to allow better focus on relaxation.

He or she can also assure others that some time out is needed to relax and that everything is under control.

Music in the Rehabilitation of Chronic Obstructive Pulmonary Disease

Research supports physical exercise as an essential component of pulmonary rehabilitation aimed at decreased dyspnea (breathing distress), health-related quality of life, and exercise tolerance in persons who have chronic lung disease, and walking helps to maintain therapeutic gains (Heppner, Morgan, Kaplan, & Ries, 2006). As with any exercise program, adherence is important to outcomes.

In an effort to support a walking program for persons with COPD, researchers studied the effect of music listening on dypsnea and anxiety while walking. The results indicated positive impressions from the music, but no statistically significant differences in dypsnea or anxiety perceptions whether or not music was heard during 10-minute walks (Brooks, Sidani, Graydon, McBride, Hall, & Weinacht, 2003). This result is not surprising since the design of the music and the walking pace are likely essential to outcomes. The music in this study was not calibrated in tempo to the walking cadence of each individual but merely consisted of music persons preferred.

In one innovative program for persons confined to bed with severe, end-stage COPD, four patients participated in case study research in which rhythmic and musical cues were used to enhance endurance and to manage exertional dyspnea (Chen, 2004). The patients had such severe physical impairments that they were admitted to the hospital for palliative, end-of-life care. Music therapists worked with a physical therapist to design the pulmonary rehabilitation program that was comprised of two parts: (1) rhythmic auditory stimulation (RAS) to slow the walking cadence, or tempo, as a way to extend the distance walked (endurance); and (2) respiratory cueing designed to facilitate pursed-lip breathing in exhalations twice as long as inhalations immediately after the walk. Breathing cues continued to gradually slow and deepen the breathing. The results of this case study research demonstrated that the patients increased their walking distance from one to two steps to 80 to 120 meters in one walking bout. As their distance increased over time, several outcomes were consistent for all four patients: (1) needs for supplemental oxygen did not increase as distance increased, (2) recovery times from dypsnea following walking bouts did not increase, and (3)) the recovery times after walking required for oxygen saturation levels and heart rates to return to pre-walk levels did not increase. These patients, who reported upon admission to the program that turning over in bed required great effort and walking unassisted across the room to the bathroom was nearly impossible, were amazed and delighted with their restored functions. Though they remained on supplemental oxygen, they participated in activities within their families and within their communities, including going out to eat, shopping, getting together with friends, and participating in other activities important to them.

Two recent patients with COPD who participated in the music cued pulmonary rehabilitation protocol had functional outcomes similar to those of patients in the case study. As a result, they returned to their respective homes, rather than going to the residential nursing care placement that was planned for them upon their initial admission to the medical center.

In a study of patients with less severe COPD, a music therapy program was designed with singing instruction as the treatment (Engen, 2005). Results demonstrated that functional outcomes improved significantly. These included better breath management and better breath support that resulted in greater speech intensity. Breathing shifted from clavicular to diaphragmatic breaths that were maintained up to 2 weeks following the end of treatment.

Results of the Chen (2004) and Engen (2005) studies demonstrate the potential efficacy of rhythmic cueing, respiratory cueing, and therapeutic singing in pulmonary rehabilitation for persons who have COPD. Additional research with larger numbers of participants is necessary to confirm the outcomes and to explain their contributions to life quality for persons who have COPD.

MUSIC AND RELIEF OF NAUSEA AND VOMITING RESULTING FROM CHEMOTHERAPY

The use of chemotherapy in the treatment of cancer carries with it many side effects, including nausea and vomiting. Vomiting can be so severe that it can result in bone fractures, esophageal tissue tears, eating disturbances, metabolic disorders, and other serious consequences (Tipton et al., 2007). The vomiting associated with chemotherapy is so disturbing to cancer patients that 25–50% of them postpone their treatments (Lazio, 1983) and 10% terminate their series of treatments prematurely (Siegel & Longo, 1981).

Nausea and vomiting can be managed using medications. These medications are selected for their particular effectiveness with certain drugs, the route and duration of their administration, and the dosage given (Wilkes, 1991). Even with pharmacological intervention, elimination of vomiting may require several trials in order to find the best schedule and the best combination of drugs, and vomiting may occur during the course of the trials.

Even when complete pharmacological management is achieved during treatment, people receiving chemotherapy may experience anticipatory nausea and vomiting as the time for their next round of therapy approaches (Roscoe et al., 2004). This response is the result of fear and anxiety, not an actual response to chemical agents. People may become nauseated enough to vomit at the mere thought of their next treatment or when they encounter certain sounds, smells, people, or other stimuli that they associate with chemotherapy.

Anticipatory nausea and vomiting may be managed by diverting attention from the triggering stimuli and by reducing the associated anxiety and fear. Research indicates that management can be achieved by listening to music alone or by combining it with relaxation techniques (Ferrer, 2005; Fiore, 2004; Frank, 1985; Standley, 1992). Effectiveness depends largely upon early implementation and practice at times of no discomfort so that relaxation responses and attention diversion techniques can be accessed readily. (See Appendices for relaxation approaches with music.)

At the first wave of nausea, individuals must take slow, deep breaths and begin their relaxation technique as they activate, either mechanically or mentally, their preselected relaxation music. This music must fit the individual's musical taste, be very familiar, and calm the person. The relaxation technique is performed while sitting in a comfortable, somewhat reclined position, with the head and upper body well elevated. It is important for the nauseous person to remain upright because lying down may stimulate a vomiting response.

If vomiting should occur, the danger of blocking the airway or aspirating vomitus into the lungs is increased.

The focus of attention on music and on the relaxation technique of choice can block the sensations of nausea. Music and relaxation techniques can provide a viable, effective approach to self-management and control of anticipatory nausea that may occur in people in chemotherapy.

CONCLUSION

The use of music and relaxation techniques is viable in managing physical stress and discomfort and the anxieties and fears associated with them. The techniques are relatively simple, easy to learn, and accessible to most people. Their effectiveness depends on continual practice. The techniques may require some adjustments in order to meet the special needs of people who wish to use them. In addition, total effectiveness may be realized only after consultation with a music therapist, who is trained to design and implement therapeutic music approaches to manage pain and discomfort.

REFERENCES

Aldwin, C. M., & Werner, E. E. (2007). *Stress, coping, and development: An integrative perspective* (2nd ed.). New York: Guilford Press.

Almerud, S., & Petersson, K. (2003). Music therapy—A complementary treatment for mechanically ventilated intensive care patients. *Intensive and Critical Care Nursing*, 19(1), 21–30.

Baker, K. B., & Kim, J. J. (2004). Amygdala lateralization in fear conditioning: Evidence for greater involvement of the right amygdala. *Behavioral Neuroscience*, 118(1), 15–23.

Bartlett, D., Kaufman, D., & Smeltekop, R. (1993). The effects of music listening and perceived sensory experiences on the immune system as measured by interleukin-1 and cortisol. *Journal of Music Therapy*, 30(4), 194–209.

Benson, H. (1992). *The relaxation response*. New York: Wings' Books.

Benson, H., & Klipper, M. Z. (2000). *The relaxation response*. New York: Harper Paperbacks.

Blonna, R. (2006). *Coping with stress in a changing world*. Columbus, OH: McGraw Hill Humanities.

Blood, A. J., & Zatorre, R. J. (2001). Intensely pleasurable responses to music correlate with activity in brain regions implicated in reward and emotion. *Proceedings of the National Academy of Science*, 98(20), 11818–11823.

Bloom, F. E., Lazerson, A., & Nelson, C. (2005). *Brain, mind and behavior* (3rd ed.). Basingstoke, Hampshire, England: Palgrave Macmillan.

Brooks, D., Sidani, S., Graydon, J., McBride, S., Hall, L., &

Weinacht, K. (2003). Evaluating the effects of music on dyspnea during exercise in individuals with chronic obstructive pulmonary disease: a pilot study. *Rehabilitation Nursing*, 28(6), 192–196.

Bruscia, K. E., & Grocke, D. E. (2002). *Guided Imagery and Music: The Bonny Method and beyond*. Gilsum, NH: Barcelona.

Carrasquillo Y., & Gereau, R. W., IV. (2007). Activation of the extracellular signal-regulated kinase in the amygdale modulates pain perception. *Journal of Neuroscience*, 27(7), 1543–1551.

Chen, Y. L. (2004). *The effects of music enhanced physical therapy treatments on endurance, management of exertional dyspnea, and perceived health status in persons with chronic obstructive pulmonary disease (COPD)*. Unpublished master's thesis, The University of Kansas, Lawrence.

Clayton, D. (1995, August). *The effect of music therapy on pain management with persons who are burned severely*. Unpublished raw data.

Davis-Rollans, C., & Cunningham, S. (1987). Physiological responses of coronary care patients to selected music. *Heart & Lung: The Journal of Critical Care*, 16(4), 370–378.

Engen, R. (2005). The singer's breath: Implications for treatment of persons with emphysema. *Journal of Music Therapy*, 42(1), 20–48.

Ferrer, A. J. (2005). *The effect of live music on decreasing anxiety in patients undergoing chemotherapy treatment*. Unpublished master's thesis, Florida State University, Tallahassee.

Fiore, J. M. (2004). *The effect of music, music and relaxation, and relaxation on chemotherapy related anxiety and nausea*. Unpublished master's thesis, University of Kansas, Lawrence.

Frank, J. (1985). The effects of music therapy and guided visual imagery on chemotherapy-induced nausea and vomiting. *Oncology Nursing Forum*, 12(5), 47–52.

Fratianne, R. B., Presner, J. D., Huston, M. J., Super, D. M., Yowler, C. J., & Standley, J. M. (2001). The effect of music-based imagery and musical alternate engagement on the burn debridement process. *Journal of Burn Care and Rehabilitation*, 22(1), 47–53.

Gosselink, R. (2004). Breathing techniques in patients with chronic obstructive pulmonary disease (COPD). *Chronic Respiratory Disease*, 1(3), 163–172.

Guzzetta, C. (1989). Effects of relaxation and music therapy on patients in a coronary care unit with presumptive acute myocardial infarction. *Heart & Lung: The Journal of Critical Care*, 18(6), 609–616.

Heppner, P. S., Morgan, C., Kaplan, R. M., & Ries, A. L. (2006). Regular walking and long-term maintenance of outcomes after pulmonary rehabilitation. *Journal of Cardiopulmonary Rehabilitation*, 26(1), 44–53.

Hirokawa, E., & Ohira, H. (2003). The effects of music listening after a stressful task on immune functions, neuroendocrine responses, and emotional states in college students. *Journal of Music Therapy*, 40(3), 189–211.

Hucklebridge, F., Lambert, S., Clow, A., Awarburton, D. M., Evans, P. D., & Sherwood, N. (2000). Modulation of secretory immunoglobulin A in saliva: Response to manipulation of mood. *Biological Psychology*, 53(1), 25–35.

Ikeda, R., Takahashi, Y., Kazuhine, I., & Kato, F. (2007). NMDA receptor-independent synaptic plasticity in the central amygdala in the rat model of neuropathic pain. *Pain*, 127 (1–2), 161–172.

Jacobson, E. (1938). *Progressive relaxation*. Chicago: University of Chicago Press.

Ji, G., Fu, Y., Ruppert, K. A., Neugebauer, V. (2007). Pain-related anxiety-like behavior requires CRF1 receptors in the amygdala. *Molecular Pain*, 3, 13.

Ji, G., & Neugebauer, V. (2007). Differential effects of CRF1 and CRF2 receptor antagonists on pain-related sensitization of neurons in the central nucleus of the amygdale. *Journal of Neurophysiology*, 97(6), 3893–3904.

Koelsch, S., Fritz, T. V., Cramon, D. Y., Müller, K., & Friederici, A. D. (2006). Investigating emotion with music: An FMRI study. *Human Brain Mapping*, 27(3), 239–250.

Korn, E. R. (1983). The use of altered states of consciousness and imagery in physical and pain rehabilitation. *Journal of Mental Imagery*, 7(1), 25–34.

Kwentus, J., Harkins, S., Lignon, N., & Silverman, J. (1985). Current concepts of geriatric pain and its treatment. *Geriatrics*, 40(4), 48–54, 57.

Lazio, J. (1983). Nausea and vomiting as major complications of cancer chemotherapy. *Drugs*, 25(Suppl. 1), 1–7.

Leuner, H. (1978). Basic principles and therapeutic efficacy of guided affective imagery. In J. L. Singer, & K. S. Pope (Eds.), *The power of human imagination* (pp. 125–166). New York: Plenum Press.

Malseed, R. T., Goldstein, F. J., & Balkon, N. (1995). *Pharmacology: Drug therapy and nursing considerations* (4th ed.). Philadelphia: Lippincott Williams & Wilkins.

McCaffery, M., & Pasero, C. (1999). *Pain: Clinical manual* (2nd ed.). St. Louis, MO: Mosby.

McDermott, F., & O'Callaghan, C. (2004). Music therapy's relevance in a cancer hospital researched through a constructivist lens. *Journal of Music Therapy*, 41(2), 151–185.

Miller, D. (1992). *The effect of music therapy on the immune and adrenocortical systems of cancer patients.* Unpublished master's thesis, University of Kansas, Lawrence.

Minois, N. (2000). Longevity and aging: Beneficial effects of exposure to mild stress. *Biogerontolgy*, 1(1), 15–29.

Neugebauer, V. (2004). The amygdala and persistent pain. *The Neuroscientist*, 10(3), 221–234.

Neugebauer, V. (2007). The amygdala: Different pains, different mechanisms. *Pain*, 127(1–2), 161–172.

Neupert, S. D., Almedia, D. M., & Charles, S. T. (2007). Age differences in reactivity to daily stressors: The role of personal control. *The Journals of Gerontology Series B: Psychological Sciences and Social Sciences*, 6(4), 216–225.

O'Sullivan, R. (1991). A music road to recovery: Music in intensive care. *Intensive Care Nursing*, 7(3), 160–163.

Pedersen, L. H., Scheel-Krüger, J., & Blackburn-Munro G. (2007, January). Amygdala GAVA-A receptor involvement in mediating sensory-discriminative and affective-motivational pain responses in a rat model of peripheral nerve injury. *Pain*, 127(1–2), 17–26.

Powers, P. S., Cruse, C. W., Daniels, S., & Stevens, B. (1994). Post-traumatic stress disorder in patients with burns. *Journal of Burn Care and Rehabilitation*, 15(2), 147–153.

Presner, J. D., Yowler, C. J., Smith, L. F., Steele, A. L., & Fratianne, R. B. (2001). Music therapy for assistance with pain and anxiety management in burn treatment. *Journal of Burn Care and*

Rehabilitation, 22(1), 83–88.

Rider, M., Achterberg, J., Lawlis, G., Goven, A., Toledo, R., & Butler, J. (1990). Effect of immune system imagery on secretory IgA. *Biofeedback and Self-Regulation*, 15(4), 317–333.

Robb, S. L. (2000). Music assisted progressive muscle relaxation, progressive muscle relaxation, music listening, and silence: A comparison of relaxation techniques. *Journal of Music Therapy*, 37(1), 2–21.

Rodin, J. (1986). Aging and health: Effects of the sense of control. *Science*, 233(4770), 1271.

Roscoe, J. A., Bushnow, P., Morrow, G. R., Hickok, J. T., Kuebler, P. J., Jacobs, A., & Banerjee, T. K. (2004). Patient expectation is a strong predictor of severe nausea after chemotherapy. *Cancer,* 101(11), 2701–2708.

Schober, M., & Affara, F. (2006). *Advanced practice nursing.* Oxford, England: Blackwell.

Schultz, J. H., & Luthe, W. (1969). *Autogenic therapy: Autogenic methods* (Vol. 1). New York: Grune & Stratton.

Selye, H. (1956). *The stress of life.* New York: McGraw-Hill.

Siegel, L. J., & Longo, D. L. (1981). The control of chemotherapy induced emesis. *Annals of Internal Medicine*, 95(3), 352–359.

Sin, D. D., McAlister, F. A., Man, P., & Anthonisen, N. R. (2003). Contemporary management of chronic obstructive pulmonary disease. *Journal of the American Medical Association*, 290(17), 2301–2312.

Snyder, M. (1992). *Independent nursing interventions* (2nd ed.). Albany, NY: Delmar.

Standley, J. (1992). Clinical applications of music and chemotherapy: The effects of nausea and emesis. *Music Therapy Perspectives*, 10(1), 27–35.

Tipton, J. M., McDaniel, R. W., Barbour, L., Johnston, M. P., Kayne, M., LeRoy, P., & Ripple, M. L. (2007). Putting evidence into practice: Evidence-based interventions to prevent, manage, and treat chemotherapy-induced nausea and vomiting. *Clinical Journal of Oncology Nursing*, 11(1), 1092–1095.

Tsao, C., Gordon, T., Maranto, D., Lerman, C., & Murasko, D. (1991). The effects of music and biological imagery on immune response (s-Iga). In C. D. Maranto (Ed.), *Application of music in medicine* (pp. 85–121). Washington, DC: National Association for Music Therapy.

Updike, P. (1990). Music therapy results for ICU patients. *Dimensions of Critical Care Nursing*, 9(1), 39–45.

Urden, L. D., Stacy, K. M., & Lough, M. E. (2005). *Thelan's critical care nursing: Diagnosis and management* (5th ed.). St. Louis, MO: Mosby.

U.S. Cancer Statistics Working Group. (2007). *United States Cancer Statistics: 2003 Incidence and Mortality*. Atlanta, GA: Department of Health and Human Services, Centers for Disease Control and Prevention, and National Cancer Institute.

Voss, J., Good, M., Yates, B., Baun, M., Thompson, A., & Hertzog, M. (2004). Sedative music reduces anxiety and pain during chair rest after open-heart surgery. *Pain*, 112(1–2), 197–203.

White, J. (1992). Music therapy: An intervention to reduce anxiety in the myocardial infarction patient. *Clinical Nurse Specialist*, 6(1), 58–63.

Whitehead-Pleaux, A. M., Baryza, M. J., & Sheridan, R. L. (2006). The effects of music therapy on pediatric patients' pain and anxiety during donor site dressing change. *Journal of Music Therapy*, 43(2), 136–153.

Wilkes, G. (1991). Potential toxicities and nursing management. In M. Burke, G. Wilkes, D. Berg, C. Bean, & K. Ingwersen (Eds.), *Cancer chemotherapy: A nursing process approach* (pp. 49–138). Boston: Jones & Bartlett.

Wilkins, M. K., & Moore, M. L. (2004). Music intervention in the intensive care unit: A complementary therapy to improve patient outcomes. *Evidence-Based Nursing*, 7(4), 103–104.

Zhan, C., Sangl, J., Bierman, A., Miller, M., Friedman, B., Wickizer, S., & Meyer, G. S. (2001). Potentially inappropriate medication use in the community-dwelling elderly: Findings from the 1996 medical expenditure panel survey. *Journal of the American Medical Association*, 286(22), 2823–2829.

Chapter 6

Music to Facilitate Physical Exercise in Older Adults

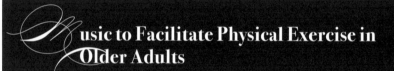
Music to Facilitate Physical Exercise in Older Adults

Music can provide stimulation and promote movement or other physical activity. Music has always been used in the background of physical activity, but it has been only since the mid-1980s that the effects of music on physical activity, the uses of music in exercise, and the importance of exercise in older adults have been studied.

IMPORTANCE OF PHYSICAL EXERCISE

Research demonstrates that those older adults who maintain active lifestyle habits into late years reduce potential disabilities or compress them into a shorter period toward the end of life. Consequently, older adults with active lifestyles have less overall lifetime disability than those who are more sedentary (Hubert, Bloch, Oehlert, & Fries, 2002; Leveille, Guralnik, Ferrucci, & Langlois, 1999).

No matter what one's age, it is essential to participate regularly in physical exercise to maximize health. However, the duration and intensity of appropriate exercise depends upon physical strength and abilities. Sitting or lying down, even for several days, leads to loss of physical abilities and organ function and to diminishing health. Thus, one of the cardinal principles of quality of life for older adults is the preservation and restoration of physical function (McAuley, Elavsky, Jerome, Konopack, & Marquez, 2005; Mihalko & McAuley, 1996; Rejeski & Mihalko, 2001; Reuben, Laliberte, Hiris, & Mor, 1990). Good physical function allows one to maintain as much independence as possible, which contributes to personal dignity. Furthermore, good physical function and the accompanying physical health are integral to mental, emotional, and social well-being, all of which contribute to opportunities that enhance the quality of life (Ellingson & Conn, 2000; Netz, Wu, Becker, & Tenenbaum, 2005).

Traditionally, bed rest was considered central to restoring health in anyone who was ill or injured. However, the shortages of hospital beds and personnel during World War II and, since the 1980s, health care cost containment made extensive bed rest impossible (Corcoran, 1991). The surprising results were improved outcomes and fewer complications with early mobilization in sick and injured people (Corcoran, 1991). Research has shown that physical disabilities worsen with bed rest (Gill, Allore, & Guo, 2004). Physical disabilities include the following:

1. Decreased range of motion and contractures

2. Disuse atrophy in muscles (Kortebein, Ferrando, Lombeida, & Wolfe, 2007)

3. Osteoporosis and bone fractures

4. Calculus formation (formation of a hard mass of mineral salts around organic material) and urinary tract infections

5. Increased heart rate with decreased number of pulse beats, threat of pulmonary embolism (obstruction of a pulmonary artery, caused by detached blood clots from a leg or pelvic vein), and orthostatic, or postural, hypotension (lowered blood pressure when rising from a lying position)

6. Atelectasis (collapse of lung tissue) and pneumonia

7. Anorexia, constipation, and malnutrition

8. Breakdown of skin, leading to bedsores

9. Sensory deprivation, which causes anxiety, hostility, depression, disorientation, and altered sleep patterns (Corcoran, 1991; Harper & Lyles, 1988)

10. Potential for chronic pain (Corcoran, 1991).

The psychosocial effects of immobility include the following (Miller, 1975):

1. Fear and panic

2. Social withdrawal

3. Apathy

4. Exacerbation of preexisting symptoms related to dementia or to other psychiatric diagnoses

5. Stupor so severe that it presents as a semicomatose state.

Age-related musculoskeletal changes that result in losses of strength and flexibility along with alterations in posture, balance, gait, and perceptions of discomfort lead to problems with mobility in older adults (Lewis, 1985). As a consequence of these and other age-related physical changes, range of motion becomes limited and a person's ability to function in the environment can be compromised (Holohan-Bell & Brummel-Smith, 1999). This ability to function is defined by each person's skills and abilities and by the requirements of his or her environment and the amounts and types of support available there (Holohan-Bell & Brummel-Smith, 1999). Therefore, a complete assessment of each individual's skills, abilities, and potential for development is required within the context of the environment in which he or she is living or wishes to live. The story of Mrs. Mackenzie illustrates how adjustments in environment and lifestyle can contribute to health and independence:

> Mrs. Mackenzie had lived alone in her own home for 20 years after the death of her husband, and she wanted to remain there for as long as possible. She was, however, beginning to experience occasional dizziness while using the stairs to the basement laundry room and to her bedroom on the second floor of the house. In addition, cooking was becoming such a difficult chore that she had resorted to a diet that consisted mainly of cold cereal and fried egg sandwiches.
>
> Although Mrs. Mackenzie was taking medication for hypertension, which managed her dizziness reasonably well, she was tempted to sit and read or watch television for most of her day. It was clear that she would lose her ability to function at home if physical and environmental interventions were not initiated. Her physician became concerned about her lack of activity and her apparent lethargy during an office visit in which she complained of feeling "blah" and of being unable to do much for herself. After completing blood work and a thorough physical exam, Mrs. Mackenzie's physician requested that the local home health care service send a staff member to Mrs. Mackenzie's residence to provide guidance in adapting her home environment to meet her physical needs. Because Mrs. Mackenzie said she "wanted more than anything in this world" to remain at home, she was extremely motivated to work with home health care staff to make the

necessary changes in her daily routine that would help her to maintain her functional abilities for as long as possible.

At the urging of the home health nurse, who was concerned about Mrs. Mackenzie's nutrition and physical flexibility, Mrs. Mackenzie joined a water aerobics class for older adults at the local parks and recreation facility, where she exercised at her capacity for 40 minutes, 3 times each week. The exercises were designed by an exercise physiologist who specialized in programs for older adults, and adaptations were made for Mrs. Mackenzie in order to make her exercise program compatible with her medication and strength needs. The exercises were accompanied by music recordings that Mrs. Mackenzie said made her feel like dancing and motivated her to exercise. To her amazement, she found the exercise classes so enjoyable that they did not seem like work at all, and she looked forward to her classes and to seeing other acquaintances there. One of the people in the class had become a special friend with whom she had coffee one day each week when the class did not meet. Mrs. Mackenzie said she began to look forward to getting out of bed in the morning, and she lost the urge to lie down to watch television for several hours during the day.

Mrs. Mackenzie is fortunate that she had access to resources in her community that provided interventions to develop her physical functioning and made it possible for her to remain in her own home. Evidence exists that such interventions in physical functioning can be successful for a wide range of older adults, even if they experience physical deterioration as a result of the process of normal aging. Posner et al. (1992) found that people who ranged in age from 60 to 86 and who were previously sedentary gained significant beneficial results after only 4 months of aerobic exercise, 3 times weekly, for 40 minutes. A comparison between people who exercised and a control group of comparable people who met weekly for 1 hour of conversation and social contact showed significant differences between the two groups. People who exercised had decreased blood pressure, increased ventilation threshold, increased physical workload, and improved oxygen uptake compared to people who did not exercise. In addition, fewer people dropped out of the exercise group than out of the control group. After 2 years, a follow-up study revealed that the exercise group had a significantly lower number of diagnoses of recent-onset cardiovascular disease than did the control group, indicating that the exercise had long-term, positive effects. These effects also held for people who exercised regularly over the 2 years as well as for people who discontinued their exercise programs after the 4-month study was completed.

Another study showed the efficacy of exercise in older people in their ability to remain independent. In a group of 687 older adults, 42.5% participated in regular exercise programs. When compared to nonexercisers, these individuals traveled without assistance more frequently, rated their perceptions of personal health more highly, scored higher on mental health index scores, and experienced lower mortality rates during a 1-year follow-up period (Reuben et al., 1990). Recent similar studies support these findings (Colcombe & Kramer, 2003; Evans, Goodman, & Redfern, 2003; LIFE Study Investigators, 2006).

Although exercise is essential for older adults, exercise programs for older people must be designed to address their special needs. Older people differ markedly from younger people in their susceptibility to the adverse effects of deconditioning that result from the greater degree of age-related physical decline and diminished physical reserves (Means, Currie, & Gershkoff, 1993). It is, therefore, essential that older adults undergo comprehensive medical examinations and physical evaluations before they begin an exercise program, and that such programs be supervised by experts who are trained to recognize indications of the negative effects of exercise, particularly on older adults. One effect is overheating (excessive body temperature), which can result in heat stress, heat cramps, heat exhaustion, and heat stroke. These conditions are managed by drinking water before exercise, by drinking 6–8 ounces of water every 15 minutes during exercise, and by wearing proper clothing during exercise (Eiserman, 1986; Evans, 1999). Other negative effects of exercise can be managed by waiting to exercise from 30 minutes to 1 hour after meals and by beginning the exercise routine with gentle warm-up stretches, continuing with moderate increases in activity, and ending gradually

(Evans, 1999; Simpson, 1986).

Older people can experience negative reactions to exercise while they are taking certain medications, such as beta blockers, which decrease the heart rate; antihypertensives, which react to exercise by magnifying the effects of the drug; and antidepressants and neuroleptics, which can produce changes in blood pressure. These people should be monitored (Simpson, 1986). Other undesirable effects of exercise include fatigue, weakness, depression, confusion, dizziness, vertigo, ataxia (an inability to coordinate voluntary muscular movement), and urinary incontinence (Chapron & Besdine, 1986).

The positive effects of exercise on quality of life are such that exercise should be attempted, at least for a short time, even by physically frail older adults (Holohan-Bell & Brummel-Smith, 1999). Their reactions to exercise can be monitored so that detrimental effects can be avoided. Other less frail older people can learn the warning signs of overexertion or impending physical injury and can learn to monitor their own reactions to exercise, both positive and negative. They can also learn how much and what types of activity are best for them, and when to curb their usual exercise routines.

USING MUSIC DURING PHYSICAL EXERCISE

Role of Music in Adherence to Exercise

Based on the results from several recent research studies, there are strong indications that music facilitates a person's adherence to an exercise program (Elliott, Carr, & Savage, 2004; Harmon & Kravitz, 2007; Johnson, Otto, & Clair, 2001). Adherence is essential for developing and maintaining physical strength and agility; intermittent participation in exercise will not yield the desired results (Mailloux, Finno, & Rainville, 2006). Most information concerning the value of music in exercise is anecdotal. Many people report that music helps them get through their exercise program and that without music, the program seems to last longer than it actually does. They also report that music seems to help them to push themselves further, to remain in the program, and to look forward to their exercise sessions.

A study of 30 college students (15 male, 15 female) has supported some of these anecdotal reports. When these college students participated in an aerobic walking program that used music continually, used it intermittently, and did not use music at all, they walked significantly farther with music than they did without it (Beckett, 1990). Although no statistically significant differences were found between listening to music continually and listening to it intermittently, there were some indications that intermittent music was more effective than continual music in producing increased distances. In addition, the students had faster heart rate recoveries following exercise with both continual and intermittent music than they had with no music, and they walked farther with less effort with music than they did without it. It should be noted that each of the subjects was tested individually, and subjects served as their own controls. Subjects also chose their own music and selected the volume at which it was played for each exercise session.

Regular involvement in an exercise regimen is difficult for older people who experience physical discomfort and have additional problems with confusion (Mathews, Clair, & Kosloski, 2001). Research at the University of Kansas (Terasaki, 1993) tested the feasibility of using (1) musical instrument playing, (2) background music, (3) metronome clicks, and (4) no music during regularly scheduled physical therapy sessions that were designed to maintain the upper body range of motion in a group of residents in a nursing facility. Terasaki's results indicated that playing a musical instrument and background music, incorporated into a regular exercise regimen, did not significantly increase range of motion from pretest to posttest, and that range of motion was not significantly greater in people exercising to the accompaniment of a musical instrument than it was in people who exercised without the playing of a musical instrument or background music or in people who did not use music in their exercise regimens. Terasaki's study was limited, however, by the size of the subject sample, which decreased from 36 to 25 participants over the course of 8 weeks. Although the 25 subjects were assigned randomly to each of the four musical conditions, insufficient numbers of participants in the study likely influenced the results.

Terasaki observed that participants exhibited other behaviors that indicated the level of their commitment to participation. People who exercised while listening to both taped music and live music ($N = 5$)

adhered to the program throughout its 24-session duration. They often commented after an exercise session that they were amazed that the exercise session was finished for the day. These people were also quite verbal during the sessions and freely encouraged one another to participate with comments such as, "Come on, you can do it," "Don't stop now," "We're on the right track," and "Hang in there, and I will, too."

The behaviors of the people who exercised to musical instrument accompaniment were contrasted with the behaviors of people in other groups who withdrew from the exercise protocols before they were completed or who failed to complete the required number of repetitions in the regimen. These people complained of discomfort and pain throughout the exercise sessions and gave no encouragement to one another. Their affect was generally one of displeasure, and they generally greeted the therapist who conducted the sessions with, "Oh, is it time for you already? I thought we just did this yesterday. How many more times do we have to do all this?"

Terasaki's observations indicate that active participation in exercise and adherence to exercise programs may be enhanced with a music therapy intervention that motivates and supports participation through rhythmic structure and enjoyment of music. In addition, socialization and mutual support brought about by music during exercise may also contribute to positive experiences, making adherence more likely.

Exercise with Music Supports Specific Exercise Movements

A series of research studies conducted by Hamburg and Clair has demonstrated that a specifically designed movement exercise program, *Motivating Moves*, was successful in improving physical function in well older adults. Within *Motivating Moves*, Hamburg, a Laban movement analyst, designed a series of 14 exercises to facilitate physical flexibility in older adults. Each exercise in the program was cued by music that was improvised to specifically reflect the movement dynamics, number of repetitions, duration, and speed of each movement within the exercise. The music was sequenced and recorded for each of the exercises as follows: (1) a musical introduction to provide an auditory cue movement initiation; (2) music to cue the speed, range, duration, and repetitions of specific movements; (3) a clear musical ending to give an auditory cue for closure to the movement; and (4) a 3-second break between musical selections.

The outcomes of the music-cued Motivating Moves program for one study indicated improved functional skills after 5 weeks. These included statistically significant increases in Reuben's Physical Performance Test (Reuben & Siu, 1990) items of gait speed and putting on and removing a jacket (Hamburg & Clair, in press). In two earlier studies, well older adults demonstrated statistically significant increases in measures of balance and gait characteristics after five weekly sessions in the music-cued *Motivating Moves* program (Hamburg & Clair, 2003a, 2003b). Research outcomes have consistently demonstrated that the music-cued movement program *Motivating Moves* is quite successful in facilitating positive functional outcomes in populations of well older persons.

Music that Encourages Participation in Exercise

Preferences for Music

Terasaki's (1993) observations that music contributes to positive experiences that facilitate adherence to an exercise regimen not withstanding, some styles or types of music are better facilitators than others. To best encourage participation, it is important to choose music that is preferred by the person who will be using it. This preferred music is more likely to encourage participation than music that is not preferred. People associate the preferred music with pleasant experiences and/or feelings. When the music is paired with exercise, the exercise also becomes a pleasant, or at least nonaversive, experience.

Some participants may have narrow music preferences. Music selections for exercise must often include nonpreferred music in order to match the various physical activity levels required throughout an exercise session. An individual or group can listen to samples of music selected for activity level suitability in order to determine which music may be most appropriate. Music that is nonaversive, or music for which there is no dislike, may be acceptable. Trying various types of musical styles in exercise sessions is the best test of appropriateness, and a person's or a group's use of it over time can even cause a preference for it to be developed.

This developed preference, or tolerance for music not initially preferred, has been demonstrated in the results of a 1999 study designed to determine the effects of silence, most-preferred music, and least-preferred music on the participation of older men in a task. These men, physically frail residents of a U.S. Department of Veterans Affairs nursing home care unit in the Midwest, were involved in a program designed to promote upper body activity through sanding and assembling wooden toys. The certified therapeutic recreation specialist who supervised the program collaborated with the music therapists on staff to design a study that could determine changes in participation levels during silence, most-preferred background music, and least-preferred background music. When the study began, the men stopped participating upon hearing opera music, which they indicated as their least-preferred music. Not only did they stop participating in the task at hand, but they verbally expressed their dislike and displeasure concerning the unfamiliar music. Opera was not usually heard on their local radio stations or television programs, and there was little opportunity to hear it performed live. They were very familiar, however, with big band dance tunes, which they all indicated to be their preferred music. When opera was discontinued and big band music was substituted, the men resumed their tasks. After several weeks, however, their patterns of participation began to change. They continued to work without a break when opera music was played, just as they had when the big band music was used. Indications are that the men's tolerance for least-preferred music shifted over time with more exposure to it, and that they may have begun to develop a liking for it. They no longer reacted negatively to the music they once indicated as their least preferred (Otto, Cochran, Johnson, & Clair, 1999).

Based on the results from this study, there are strong indicators that nonpreferred music can become music that facilitates participation in activities when used over time. This may be particularly true when the experience is positive. In the case of the Otto, Cochran, Johnson and Clair study, the participants met once a week to do some valued work that they had enjoyed previously in their lives. The outcome of their labor was toys that were accepted by the U.S. Marines in their Toys for Tots program for distribution over the winter holidays to children in the community. These veterans experienced camaraderie with one another during their work sessions. They were also pleased that the products of their labors would add to the delight of young children and that their contributions to the community were acknowledged by the military. The program sessions were very positive and enjoyable, as were all associations with them, including music previously considered distasteful.

Choices of Music for Exercise

Although preferred music is best for many applications, it is not necessarily appropriate for all exercise activities. The beat of the music must fit the rate at which a particular activity is conducted and must fit the portion of the session in which it is included (Mathews et al., 2001). Therefore, a gradual warm-up to stretch the muscles at the beginning of each exercise session should include musical selections that are slow in tempo. These selections may include string or woodwind instruments and should have little syncopation and only slightly accented beats. As the stretches are completed and the repetitive movements begin, the tempo of the music should increase. The music should also have clearly heard beats that are embellished by percussion instruments. As the exercise progresses, music must continue to stimulate muscle activity through tempos matched to the repetition rate that is best suited to the individual (Karageorghis, Jones, & Low, 2006). Regardless of tempo, the music must have sufficient rhythmic qualities to stimulate continued participation.

When the exercise activity is completed, music that is appropriate to the cool-down portion of the session should be played. The cool-down begins with a decreased pace of movement. As with the warm-up period, the music in the cool-down period is slower, with rhythmic beats that facilitate continued participation. As the activity gradually winds down, so does the music. The session ends with slow stretches, accompanied by unaccented music and slow tempos. Although this music is of the same type used for the warm-up period, it should probably be made up of different selections so that participation is associated with the end, and not the beginning, of the session. As this music plays and the session comes to an end, participants move into a relaxation period. This relaxation period can last for as little as 5 minutes or can be extended to any desirable and practical amount of time. Regardless of duration, this time is designed to allow enjoyment of the relaxed state brought about through exercise. Slow, meditative-type music is used to facilitate it. This music should be characterized by unaccented beats and a very slow tempo. Harp, violin, guitar, or flute music or music performed on a synthesizer can be used. Some people may prefer to use inspirational music, which may include vocals.

During the exercise session, adherence to the program can be encouraged by providing guidance to the participants about how to make the music work for them. The participants who cannot keep the pace and maintain their heart rate within their target zone or who cannot keep pace with the tempo of the music for other reasons may not know how to adapt their participation to fit the music. Consequently, they may withdraw from the program. Exercise instructors can help by demonstrating how movements can be done in half time or even whole time for each beat pattern, which is generally based on four beat pulses per pattern. That is, when the pace requires a movement during each beat, people who must move more slowly might participate by making one movement every two beats. For people who must participate at even slower rates, one movement every four beats or one movement in as many beats as necessary while remaining in the rhythmic structure may be possible. Although people who use the slower movements make fewer repetitions than people who can maintain one movement per beat, they are able to participate. As they participate, they move with the structure of the rhythmic beats rather than struggle against them. Consequently, their experience with the music is positive and facilitative, and they are more likely to adhere to a regular schedule.

Volume of Music

Once the style of music is selected and the music matched to the type of activity, consensus must be reached concerning the volume of the music. There is no evidence that very loud music does more to motivate and encourage exercise participation than music played at a moderate volume. Loud music may also be contraindicated, especially if music blocks physical discomfort. With such blocks some people may not be as capable of monitoring their physical responses, which could put them at risk. Loud music is especially uncomfortable for people who have little or no experience with it, and it can be detrimental to people who have some hearing loss and wear hearing aids. Loud music also makes it difficult to hear the group leader's instructions. (Exercise group leaders may suffer serious vocal strain, which can lead to long-term damage to their voices.) Consequently, the most appropriate volume of music in exercise should be determined by the people using it. The level must be comfortable. Though a comfortable level is easily determined by individuals using headphones, consensus must be reached in an exercise group or class.

For example, music is often used in health clubs and recreation facilities to accompany individual exercise programs that use stair machines, weight machines, stationary bicycles, and other apparatus. Commonly, aerobics classes are conducted in an area alongside the machines or in an adjoining room. This music is often played at a high volume and the instructors must raise their voices above the music to provide instructions for the various moves or routines and instructions for monitoring heart rate and participating at one's own pace. Complaints made about the music by persons working outside the aerobics class are often met with response such as, "I'm sorry, but everyone else likes it. Maybe you can come at a different time of day." A review of the daily schedule usually reveals that aerobics classes are heavily scheduled throughout the day. A 56-year-old woman who was interested in regular exercise in order to prevent osteoporosis commented:

> I paid "big bucks" to belong to a women's exercise club. I was told when I initiated my year-long membership that there was a particular interest in acquiring members who were middle-aged through elderly, and that the exercise physiologist on staff would design a program just for me to help maintain bone mass, physical strength, and agility. I was quite pleased that there was such attention to persons my age and older, and I was excited to begin the program. Well, I got started. The exercise physiologist did an evaluation of my physical strength and talked to me about body fat. She and I worked together to design a program that would be something I could stick with for a good long time. She taught me how to use the

equipment and cautioned me about overuse. I learned how to monitor my heart rate and to know the signals for overheating and such. Then I began. I worked out three times a week for the first month, but the music they played in the place was so horrible that I haven't been back since. If the music did not come from an aerobics class, some young, skinny girl in the equipment room had a boom box blaring. So much for my exercise program. I really liked how good I felt after finishing my routine, but I just could not stand the noise in the place.

This woman's experience at her health club is not uncommon, whether the exercise program is offered at little or no cost as a community service or at high cost in a private club or resort. Most facilities incorporate loud, commercially produced exercise music that is characterized by strong beats, fairly fast tempos, and a pop/rock style. This recorded music may or may not include verbal cues for an exercise regimen. Some people enjoy this type of music and find it helps them to motivate themselves, whereas others find it so aversive that they withdraw from the program. These dropouts report that they love the exercise, but that they dislike the music and its loud volume.

CONCLUSION

Exercise is not enjoyable for many older people, especially when it leads to physical discomfort. However, exercise is essential to maintain health and well-being. Music can ease the undesirability and difficulty associated with exercise to help ensure consistent participation. For some people, the use of music in exercise can have such pleasant effects that it may even lead to enjoyment. Whether people learn to enjoy exercise accompanied by music or merely use music to facilitate their engagement in exercise, the positive effects can improve their quality of life.

REFERENCES

Beckett, A. (1990). The effects of music on exercise as determined by physiological recovery heart rates and distance. *Journal of Music Therapy*, 27(3), 126–136.

Chapron, D., & Besdine, R. (1986). Drugs as an obstacle to rehabilitation: A primer for therapists. *Topics in Geriatric Rehabilitation*, 2, 63–81.

Colcombe, S., & Kramer, A. F. (2003). Fitness effects on the cognitive function of older adults. *Psychological Science*, 14(2), 125–130.

Corcoran, P. J. (1991). Rehabilitation medicine adding life to years: Use it or lose it—the hazards of bed rest and inactivity. *Western Journal of Medicine*, 154(5), 536–538.

Eiserman, P. L. (1986). Hot weather, exercise, old age, and the kidneys. *Geriatrics*, 41, 108–114.

Ellingson, T., & Conn, V. S. (2000). Exercise and quality of life in elderly individuals. *Journal of Gerontological Nursing*, 26(3), 17–25.

Elliott, D., Carr, S., & Savage, D. (2004). Effects of motivational music on work output and affective responses during sub-maximal cycling of a standardized perceived intensity. *Journal of Sport Behavior*, 27(2), 134–147.

Evans, C. J., Goodman, C., & Redfern, S. (2003). Maintaining independence in the cognitively intact elderly care home population: A systematic review of intervention trials. *Reviews in Clinical Gerontology*, 13(2), 163–174.

Evans, W. J. (1999). Exercise training guidelines for the elderly. *Medicine and Science in Sports and Exercise*, 31(1), 12–17.

Gill, T. M., Allore, H., & Guo, Z. (2004). The deleterious effects of bed rest among community-living older persons. *The Journals of Gerontology Series A: Biological Sciences and Medical Sciences*, 59(7), M755–M761.

Hamburg, J., & Clair, A. A. (2003a). The effects of a Laban-based movement program with music on measures of balance and gait in older adults. *Activities, Adaptations, & Aging*, 28(1), 17–33.

Hamburg, J., & Clair, A. A. (2003b). The effects of a physical movement program on measures of balance and gait speed in healthy older adults. *Journal of Music Therapy*, 40(3), 212–226.

Hamburg, J., & Clair, A. A. (in press). The effects of a Laban/Bartenieff-based movement program with music on physical function measures in older adults. *Music Therapy Perspectives*.

Harmon, N. M., & Kravitz, L. (2007). The beat goes on: The effects of music on exercise: A review of the research on the ergogenic and psychophysical impact of music in an exercise program. *IDEA Fitness Journal*, 4(8), 72–77.

Harper, C. M., & Lyles, Y. M. (1988). Physiology and complications of bed rest. *Journal of the American Geriatric Society*, 36(11), 1047–1054.

Holohan-Bell, J. K., & Brummel-Smith, K. (1999). Impaired mobility and deconditioning. In J. T. Stone, J. F. Wyman, & S. A. Salisbury (Eds.), *Clinical gerontologial nursing: A guide to advanced practice* (2nd ed.) (pp. 267–288). Philadelphia: W. B. Saunders.

Hubert, H. B., Bloch, D. A., Oehlert, J. W., & Fries, J. F. (2002). *Lifestyle habits and compression of morbidity*, 57A, M347–M351.

Johnson, G., Otto, D., & Clair, A. A. (2001). The effect of instrumental and vocal music on adherence to a physical rehabilitation exercise program with persons who are elderly. *Journal of Music Therapy*, 38(2), 82–96.

Karageorghis, C. I., Jones, L., & Low, D. C. (2006). Relationship between exercise heart rate and music tempo preference. *Research Quarterly for Exercise and Sport*, 77(2), 240–244, 246–250.

Kortebein, P., Ferrando, A., Lombeida, J., & Wolfe, R. (2007). Effect of 10 days of bed rest on skeletal muscle in healthy older adults. *Journal of the American Medical Association*, 297(16), 1772–1774.

Leveille, S. G., Guralnik, J. M., Ferrucci, L., & Langlois, J. A. (1999). Aging successfully until death in old age: Opportunities for increasing active life expectancy. *American Journal of Epidemiology*, 149(7), 654–664.

Lewis, C. (1985). Clinical implications of museuloskeletal changes with age. In C. Lewis (Ed.), *Aging: The health care challenge* (pp. 117–140). Philadelphia: F.A. Davis.

LIFE Study Investigators. (2006). Effects of a physical activity intervention on measures of physical performance: Results of the lifestyle interventions and independence for elders pilot (LIFE-P) study. *The Journal of Gerontology Series A: Biological Sciences and Medical Sciences*, 61, 1157–1165.

Mailloux, J., Finno, M., & Rainville, J. (2006). Long-term exercise adherence in the elderly with chronic low back pain. *American Journal of Physical Medicine and Rehabilitation*, 85(2), 120-126.

Mathews, R. M., Clair, A. A., & Kosloski, K. (2001). Keeping the beat: Use of rhythmic music during exercise activities for the elderly with dementia. *American Journal of Alzheimer's Disease and Other Dementias*, 16(6), 377–380.

McAuley, E., Elavsky, S., Jerome, G. J., Konopack, J. F., & Marquez, D. X. (2005). Physical activity-related well-being in older adults: Social cognitive influences. *Psychology and Aging*, 20(2), 295–302.

Means, K. M., Currie, D. M., & Gershkoff, A. M. (1993). Geriatric rehabilitation. IV: Assessment, preservation, and enhancement of fitness and function. *Archives of Physical Medicine and Rehabilitation*, 74(5-S), S417–S420.

Mihalko, S. L., & McAuley, E. (1996). Strength training effects on subjective well-being and physical function in the elderly. *Journal of Aging and Physical Activity*, 4(1), 56–68.

Miller, M. B. (1975). Iatrogenic and nursigenic effects of prolonged immobilization of the ill aged. *Journal of the American Geriatric Society*, 23(8), 360–369.

Netz, Y., Wu, M., Becker, B. J., & Tenenbaum, G. (2005). Physical activity and psychological well-being in advanced age: A meta-analysis of intervention studies. *Psychology and Aging*, 20(2), 272–284.

Otto, D., Cochran, V. V., Johnson, G., & Clair, A. A. (1999). The influence of background music on task engagement in frail, older persons in residential care. *Journal of Music Therapy*, 36(3), 182–195.

Posner, J. D., Gorman, K. M., Windsor-Landsberg, L., Larsen, J., Bleiman, M., Shaw, C., Rosenberg, R., & Knebl, J. (1992). Low to moderate intensity endurance training in healthy older adults: Physiological responses after four months. *Journal of the American Geriatrics Society*, 40(1), 1–7.

Rejeski, W. J., & Mihalko, S. L. (2001). Physical activity and quality of life in older adults. *Journals of Gerontology*, 56A(Suppl. 2), 23–35.

Reuben, D., & Siu, A. (1990). An objective measure of physical function of elderly persons: A physical performance test. *Journal of the American Geriatric Society*, 38(10), 1105–1112.

Reuben, D. B., Laliberte, L., Hiris, J., & Mor, V. (1990). A hierarchical exercise scale to measure function at the advanced activities of daily living (AADL) level. *Journal of the American Geriatrics Society*, 38(8), 855–861.

Simpson, W. M. (1986). Exercise: Prescriptions for the elderly. *Geriatrics*, 41(1), 95–100.

Terasaki, Y. (1993). *The effect of music and exercise on elbow extension and flexion in elderly care home residents*. Unpublished master's thesis, University of Kansas, Lawrence.

Chapter 7

Therapeutic Uses of Music in Surgery, Invasive Medical Procedures, and Palliative Care

Therapeutic Uses of Music in Surgery, Invasive Medical Procedures, and Palliative Care

Music has been associated with physical healing since the beginning of civilization. As early as 5000 to 6000 B.C., music was included in magic and religious healing ceremonies, and was also integrated into "rational medicine," where it was used until "scientific medicine" began to be emphasized in the late 18th century (Davis & Gfeller, 1999). Even after the advent of scientific medicine, music was used to provide comfort during surgical procedures well into the 20th century at such institutions as Duke University Hospital (Durham, North Carolina) in 1929 and the University of Chicago Clinics in 1948 (Taylor, 1981). Research indicated increased comfort, reduced fear, and reduced need for heavy sedation before and during surgery, which resulted in more rapid recovery (Taylor, 1981). With such positive results, it is a mystery that the uses of music in surgery did not persist in the United States. Perhaps the development and use of effective sedatives and anesthesias made the use of music seem cumbersome and unnecessary. Perhaps music as an art form was considered incompatible with scientific research models and was therefore excluded from clinical research applications. Whatever the reason for the exclusion, there is renewed interest in using music as an intervention that improves care and patients' health and well-being in the medical setting. Physicians such as Bernie Siegel (1994, 1999) Larry Dossey (1993), and Mitchell Gaynor (2002) have encouraged patients to use all the medical and nonmedical resources available for relief and healing, including music and the other fine arts. Nurses have also begun to research and recognize the beneficial results of music in clinical applications with their patients (Biley, 1992; Cooke, Chaboyer, Schluter, & Hiratos, 2005; Lim & Locsin, 2006; Siedliecki & Good, 2006).

EFFECTS OF MUSIC IN MEDICAL AND DENTAL PROCEDURES

A great deal of literature documents the efficacy of music in the management of discomfort during medical and dental treatments. Standley (1986) examined the empirical studies that were published before 1985, analyzed their outcomes, and developed clinical applications of music therapy techniques and program development in the general hospital setting. This landmark study began with a comprehensive review of the literature concerning physiological and audio-analgesic laboratory studies and clinical studies of the therapeutic uses of music in medicine and dentistry. Standley included a meta-analysis of the results of these studies. These results led to the conclusion that music, either alone or in combination with other approaches, enhanced medical objectives, whether measured by physiological, psychological/self-report, or behavioral observation. Consequently, patients who heard music during a medical or dental procedure experienced less discomfort than patients who did not hear music before, during, or after medical or dental procedures.

Additionally, Standley (1992) analyzed 26 empirical studies of the actual effects of music on medical or dental treatments. The results also strongly support the effectiveness of music in the reduction of discomfort and pain. Numerous recent research studies (Good, Anderson, Stanton-Hicks, Grass, & Makii, 2002; Kenny & Faunce, 2004; Kwekkeboom, 2003; Whitehead-Pleaux, 2006) clearly indicate the efficacy of music in discomfort reduction and pain management.

A review of the literature fails to reveal whether music provides a diversional distraction from pain or discomfort, masks it, or actually blocks the neuropathways that transmit it. With less pain and/or discomfort, there is less need for sedation and anesthesia. Consequently, there is less danger of the adverse effects that accompany pharmacological intervention. In general, for the best results, music should be used in conjunction with anesthetics (Standley, 1986). It is also important to note that music is not a substitute for medical intervention.

BASIC PRINCIPLES OF MUSIC USED DURING SURGERY AND MEDICAL PROCEDURES REQUIRING ANESTHESIA

Marked changes in comfort levels are seen when music is used during invasive procedures, which include surgery and certain medical examinations and treatments (e.g., colonoscopy, bronchoscopy, burn debridement) (Maranto, 1991). In general, anesthesia is administered during these procedures, and music, when paired with relaxation techniques, can effectively enhance relief. Music predisposes patients to relax by the following methods:

1. Establishing a comfortable, familiar environment in the hospital or other medical facility

2. Initiating positive and pleasant experiences in a setting usually associated with physical pain and feelings of anxiety

3. Structuring the time patients must wait before, during, and after-procedures

4. Offering a distraction from the procedure

5. Quieting the effects of the bustling routines of the medical facility.

Music can supplement the human touch of nursing and other medical staff. Although personal attention and concern about comfort is at the heart of the care provided by medical staff, there is not enough time or staff available to continuously be with patients. Music can fill the gap between personal contacts made by medical staff before, during, and after procedures. Music, therefore, reduces patients' isolation and frees medical staff to deliver care more effectively and efficiently (Robb, 2000). Music is not a substitute for contact with professional medical staff, but it can provide structure and stability to help patients cope with discomfort and stress. As patients use music to cope, staff members can more effectively meet the real emotional and physical needs of each patient.

When patients have little or no coping strategies and their every need constitutes an emergency with intense and incessant demands for remediation, busy staff members become harried and ineffective in their care. Staff may react to demanding patients by avoiding contact with them. These patients then find themselves even more isolated. As patients' needs for attention increase as a result of fear and anxiety, their physical tension and subsequent discomfort also increase. They enter a cycle of severe distress, characterized by ever-increasing discomfort and subsequent loss of well-being. As patients fail to cope with their emotional distress, their physical discomforts increase and vice versa.

Music can help patients cope by empowering them to implement and manage certain aspects of their environment in order to enhance their level of comfort (Deng & Cassileth, 2005). This comfort is contingent upon the structure provided by music, which makes the environment predictable and secure. Familiar melodies are the same each time they are heard. Other elements of the same piece of music, including instrumentation, tonality, harmonic progression, and musical form, remain consistent throughout each hearing. With such predictability, patients can depend on stability in their environment. It is the predictability and stability of familiar music and patients' control over the use of it that reduces their anxiety, manages their discomfort, and increases their level of cooperation while they prepare for and experience medical procedures.

In addition, familiar music that is preferred has the potential to elicit physiological responses that can induce relaxation. These responses, including changes in pulse rate, blood pressure, respiration rate, and muscle tension, are related to stress and anxiety. Many studies support the influence of music on these responses, but the mixed results of the studies indicate that the influence of music is highly individualized and, therefore, is difficult to define for groups (Hodges, 1996). Physiological relaxation is incompatible with anxiety. Therefore, if an individual is physically relaxed, there is no possibility that anxiety and accompanying stress will occur (Thaut, 2005). Research has shown music to be very effective in increasing relaxation and decreasing preoperative anxiety when subjects selected their own music (Robb, Nichols, Rutan, Bishop, & Parker, 1995). Consequently, music selected by an individual because it contributes to his or her relaxation response is the appropriate music for inducing comfort, managing pain, and coping.

Coping and effective management of pain and discomfort by patients led to positive outcomes for patients, their families, and the medical staff who performed procedures (Standley, 1996, 2000). Patients who cope by using music will likely be more cooperative, and their discomfort will be less difficult to manage than for patients who do not use music. Therefore, patients who use music have more positive experiences, and their loved ones can appreciate the ease with which procedures are conducted. These positive outcomes cause staff to feel less fatigue and stress and to be able to respond to patients' actual concerns and needs, rather than merely meet their demands for attention. Staff is able to establish relationships with patients that encourage them to participate actively in their health care procedures and that promote patients' overall well-being.

Selecting Music to Use During Surgery and Medical Procedures

As with all therapeutic uses of music, it is important to consider the musical tastes and preferences of individual patients in order to select the music that will be the most effective. Music that is preferred and familiar is the most likely to produce relaxation and, subsequently, comfort–important prerequisites to discomfort and pain management. Patients who are empowered to select their own music and who use it in conjunction with relaxation and medication to effect changes in their own comfort levels respond positively to a situation in which they are otherwise helpless (Clark et al., 2006; Pelletier, 2004).

Familiar music best facilitates relaxation and relief from discomfort, unless patients have associations with the music that are not conducive to comfort. For instance, if the music triggers unpleasant memories, emotional distress, or feelings of loneliness or depression that are associated with past experiences, the music will not facilitate comfort. On the contrary, such music is likely to increase physical tension, which leads to greater physical discomfort, emotional distress, and even agitation. The best approach to determining the most effective music is to ask the patient to indicate which of several musical selections seems to be the most personally helpful, the most pleasant, and the most comforting. The selection cannot detract from their comfort level in any way.

Applying Music in Surgery and Medical Procedures

It is clear that the positive effects of music in surgery and invasive medical procedures are individualized. Consequently, presenting music in free field (a sound wave field devoid of obstacles causing reflection, diffraction, or refraction; without earphones) over a speaker system to all patients scheduled for procedures during the day is not an effective approach. Individuals may have unsettled or uncomfortable responses to music played in free field for several reasons. First, people react physically and emotionally to music, but the same or similar reactions do not occur in all people. Second, people who do not choose to have music in their environment may feel the music is an imposition. They may feel further deprived of control over a situation in which they already feel helpless. These feelings can result in agitation and physical tension. Third, the music may be associated with unpleasant experiences and therefore can be unsettling for individuals forced to listen to it.

Aversive responses to music played in free field may also be found in people who are forced to listen to commercially produced selections played in physicians' or dentists' waiting and examining rooms. This music is characterized by popular melodies that are generally arranged for string and woodwind instruments and that are played at a rather slow tempo without accented beats. The style and type of music is easily recognized, but the reformatted melodies are sometimes difficult to identify. People who are forced to hear this music often described it as "awful" or even "dreadful." However, the music, by itself, is not terrible; it is the unpleasant experiences people associate with the music that make it "awful" or "dreadful" for them. Whenever this or any other type of music is heard in conjunction with feelings of discomfort or lack of control, the music becomes as unpleasant or as disliked as the circumstance endured. Circumstances include undergoing medical procedures or examinations in a physician's office, being placed on hold on the telephone, or having teeth drilled in a dentist's chair. These experiences are generally preceded by a sometimes long waiting period. The dread of the procedure that builds during the wait while music plays in the background contributes to the negative feelings associated with the music.

One way to ensure music that has positive effects is to ask patients to bring their preferred music to the procedure and to provide some instruction about selecting music that will have the best results. The written instructions distributed to patients several weeks in advance of the procedure can also include information concerning choices of music and how to use them to "get ready." These instructions can be written in the following way:

- Select music that you really like and that makes you feel good. This music should also help you feel calm. If your procedure will take more than 1 hour, it might be best to make several selections available that help you feel calm and good. You may want to choose the specific music you want to hear at the medical facility while you wait for your procedure to begin, during your procedure, and during your recovery from anesthesia or sedation after the procedure.

- Once you find your "feel good/calming music," listen to it at home as you sit in your favorite chair or lie down. While you listen, breathe slowly and deeply. Let your shoulders drop. Be aware of any tension in your body. Practice letting go of all the tension in your body, one part at a time. Start with your face and jaws, move to your shoulders, then to your arms, followed by your hands and fingers. Next, let go of the tension in your buttocks, your thighs, your calves, and finally your feet. (You can change the sequence of body parts in order to find the one that is best for you.) Listen to the music as you let go of the tension. Continue to breathe slowly and deeply as you work through this process.

- Practice the tension-release exercise with your music as often as you can before you come in for your procedure. However, do not listen to your music while you are involved in activities, such as cooking, driving, or using power tools, as you might injure yourself if you become drowsy or inattentive. Be sure that while you do the exercise the music is helping you to relax. If you feel an increase in agitation or if the music makes you feel like you want to move around, select other music. It is important that your music work with you to help you relax and feel comfortable.

- Don't worry if pleasant thoughts come into your mind which seem to distract you while you are listening to the music. It may even be a good idea to think pleasant or comforting thoughts while you sit or lie down listening to your music, especially after all the tension is gone. If you find yourself dropping off to sleep, that's fine. Just keep the music going so that rest can become associated with it. It will feel good to be relaxed and rested before your procedure, on the day the procedure is done, and when you return home.

- Remember to bring your music and a portable, battery-powered player with headphones and fresh batteries. (Music and equipment may be provided by the medical facility. The doctor will inform you whether you should bring your own materials before your procedure.)

Once patients arrive, check in, and put on their gown for procedures, they should begin listening to their music, breathing deeply and slowly, and doing tension-release exercises. Patients should adjust the volume of their players in order to maintain focus on the music and not on the sounds and activities around them. The headphones will allow patients to listen to their music without disturbing anyone else, and they also block the sounds around them. To ensure uninterrupted listening, the portable player should have a continuous play option. If this feature is not available, a family member or a member of the nursing staff can be asked to check the player to ensure continuity.

Patients should be advised if their procedure will last longer than 1 hour. They need to prepare themselves for additional musical selections and for what should be done if the patient tires of the headphones. Patients may ask for the headphones to be removed before or after the completion of the procedure. Fatigue can result from hearing the same music repetitively, hearing music continuously, or from intolerance for headphones in place during lengthy procedures. Comfort with headphones depends on fit, experience with headphones, and interest in their use. It may be possible to use music intermittently to amplify its effects and decrease a patient's acclimation to it. Anesthetists, anesthesiologists, and nursing staff may facilitate the intermittent use of music by periodically removing and replacing headphones throughout the course of the procedure and recovery. However, it is ultimately the patients' decision whether music is continued or discontinued. Whatever they decide must be honored.

Many patients receive either an oral or intramuscular sedative as a preanesthetic for their procedure. The type, amount, and route of the anesthetic depend upon the type of procedure that is planned, the patient's age, and the patient's physical and emotional conditions. Patients who are scheduled for surgery must have their music interrupted in order to move them from their assigned room in the medical facility to the holding area for final preparation. Patients who must undergo an invasive medical procedure, such as a colonoscopy, bronchoscopy, gastrodiaphanoscopy, or heart catheterization, may or may not be moved. In some situations, these patients are placed initially in the procedure room, where they can continue listening to music once the procedure begins.

As patients are being prepared for surgery or invasive procedures, it may be necessary to remove the headphones while the patient is reminded of what is about to happen and as verification checks are made for the type and site for procedures. The music can be restored before insertion of an intravenous port through which medication can be administered, and before other readiness procedures are completed. Intravenous preanesthetic agents are generally given in the holding area, and other anesthesias that require time to take effect (e.g., spinal anesthesias, regional anesthesias) can follow. Headphones can remain in place during these procedures and while patients are transported to the operating room, moved onto the operating table, positioned for the procedure, and attached to monitoring equipment.

Using Music During Procedures Under General Anesthesia

Unless patients are to undergo procedures on their heads, faces, or necks, headphones through which music is played can remain on patients until the anesthesia is administered and consciousness is lost or throughout the procedure. Patients sometimes experience apprehension and fear in the few minutes between entering the room and the point of loss of consciousness. Music can help to reduce these feelings. If patients are well informed of what will happen during the procedure and why it must be done, they can use the information along with their music in order to cope.

Once the general anesthesia is administered, cerebral function is modified to the point that no perception of physical pain or discomfort is possible. During invasive procedures, patients receive multiple stimuli. Anesthetics alter patients' reactivity to stimuli and limit responses to them (Dripps, Eckenhoff, & Vandam, 1988). Some reactivity to environmental sounds may occur at some level, even when patients are adequately anesthetized. If this is the case, leaving patients' headphones on with their preferred music playing during procedures may have some influence on their sense of comfort and familiarity. This music can also block the conversations of medical staff and any other environmental sounds during procedures. For instance, many surgeons play music in free field while they operate. Although this music is helpful to the surgeons, patients may find it unpleasant. A simple check before procedures to ascertain whether the musical tastes of patients and their doctors or dentists are compatible will determine whether patients' headphones should be left in place or removed to allow the possible influence of the music in free field. Compatibility can be difficult to determine, however, because many patients simply say that whatever the doctor wants is fine with them. They are reluctant to assert their tastes and preferences if there is a chance that it may offend or impede their doctor's or dentist's efficiency and effectiveness. Intervention by the anesthetist, anesthesiologist, or nursing staff may help clarify the patient's taste in music so that the appropriate action can be taken by medical staff.

Using Music During Procedures Under Regional Anesthesias

Anesthesias that are defined as regional or conduction anesthesias are locally applied to block nerve impulses in order to make surgical sites impervious to pain while allowing the patient to remain fully conscious (Patt & Kaleka, 1990). Regional anesthesias include caudal (coccyx); epidural (outside the dura mater, one of the membranes that surrounds the brain and spinal cord); spinal, nerve, and field blocks; and local infiltration anesthesia (Patt & Kaleka, 1990). Generally, regional anesthesias are administered to patients outside the operating room and take effect over time. Administration of these anesthesias can cause discomfort, but management of the discomfort through relaxation techniques and distraction using music is beneficial. To reduce discomfort, patients should be allowed time to perform relaxation exercises with music before the administration of anesthesia.

After the regional anesthesia is administered, patients begin to lose sensation in the affected area, which gradually becomes completely numb. Music continues to confer familiarity and predictability to the environment as patients progressively surrender physical control to the anesthetic agent.

Once the anesthetic has reached its optimum effectiveness, patients are transferred into the operating room. Patients may choose to continue to wear their headphones throughout the procedure, provided the headphones compromise no part of the procedure. For example, if a patient is about to undergo a carotid endarterectomy, a procedure in which plaque is removed from the carotid artery in the neck, the headphones must be removed before the procedure begins as the headphones would compromise the surgeon's ability to operate on the neck. If the procedure does not involve the head or neck, patients may retain the headphones. Once patients are moved onto the operating table and placed into position, the portable player should be located within easy reach. To ensure proper fit, the headphones should be checked and adjusted following any movement of the body. To maximize effectiveness, patients must have control over the volume of their music, and the volume control must be readily available to them. Patients should practice adjusting the volume control mechanism before the procedure begins and while other activities are performed around them. This practicing increases their confidence in managing the player, diverts their attention from the staff, and ensures some element of control in a situation in which they are not in control.

At one hospital in the Midwest, patients who underwent transurethral resection of the prostate were prepped in the holding area outside the operating room. They were given a spinal block and a mild sedative that allowed them to be fully conscious during their procedures. While wearing headphones, they were moved into the operating room and onto the operating table. The music player was then placed on the chest. The arm bearing the intravenous port was restrained on an arm board and monitoring equipment was attached to it. The other arm was allowed to remain free and was folded across the chest within ready reach of the player. Often, patients rested their free hand over the compact player and placed a finger over the volume control. They were told that they could increase the volume at any time. If patients failed to make adjustments to the volume, anesthetists and anesthesiologists reminded patients that they were free to do so.

After surgery, the patients were moved into recovery for careful monitoring. They were required to remain in recovery until they could move their toes and had regained sensation to touch in their feet. In recovery, they were grouped with other postoperative patients. Music continued to play through their headphones to provide diversion from boredom and distraction from their surroundings. Some patients spent several hours in recovery before they were transported to their rooms on the surgical floor of the medical center.

Informal reports from these patients following surgery indicated that they enjoyed the music, that their procedure was stressful although not painful, and that they appreciated having the opportunities to listen to and control their music during the operation. They also liked having the music with them in the recovery room, especially because they were there for such a long time. They reported that the process, from prepping to completion, seemed to go faster than they expected and was not as bad as they thought it would be (Clair, 1987c). In general, these patients seemed to feel more comfortable than they had anticipated as a result of being distracted and having some control over the situation.

Using Music in Free Field During Procedures

When the procedure or the patient makes wearing headphones impossible, music can be played in free field, provided the surgeon, technical staff, and nursing staff do not oppose it. In general, medical personnel are responsive to any viable approach that can contribute to their patients' comfort and quick recovery. Consequently, they are not opposed to hearing the music in free field along with their patients. The music in free field used during several ophthalmic and plastic surgeries is often welcomed by surgical staff. The following unsolicited verbal reaction came from an operating room nurse (Clair, 1987b):

> You know, when we were told that a music therapist was coming to play music during surgery, I thought it was rather ridiculous. I am a big music fan, but I really didn't think music could do much here. I thought it would just be a waste because we rely on medications to manage pain and discomfort. Some medications, though, can have such serious side effects and can quickly build to toxicity levels in older patients, so we use as little as possible. Anyway, once the music therapist was here, I worried that she would get in my way while I worked, but she was careful to avoid areas where I had to move around, and she really made herself unobtrusive. I noticed that patients, particularly those who were scheduled for cataract surgeries and optical lens implants, were very calm during their surgeries, even when less sedation was used. These patients seemed to have positive experiences with mu-

sic. And a funny thing—I began to notice after a while that I wasn't so tense and didn't seem quite as tired at the end of the day. Usually I am just beat at the end of my shift. I have to remain so alert while assisting with procedures throughout the day, and standing for hours on the ceramic tiled floor gets rugged. The music, though, seemed to help me feel better, and less tired. I thought it was my imagination at first, but I really have begun to enjoy the music. I think things go better in there when music is playing.

Patients who preferred styles of music other than classical indicated that the classical music was fine, that it tended to make them feel calm, and that it did not disturb them. The music was played before surgery in the holding area, where preanesthesias were administered. The music continued as patients were given regional anesthesias and while the anesthesias took effect. When patients were moved to the operating room, music was initiated upon their entry and was continued until the procedure was completed. Volumes were adjusted for the comfort of the patients and the staff. The music was loud enough to be clearly audible, although still allowing the staff to understand the surgeon's verbal directives spoken in a quiet tone of voice.

When these patients were asked to comment on the music used in their procedures, they indicated that they liked it. Patients reported that they remembered hearing the music when the surgery began, but as the procedure continued, they either did not notice or they hardly noticed it. The music seemed to fade into the background. They experienced little or no discomfort throughout their procedures. They also observed that the procedure did not seem to take as long as they though it would and that it was a more pleasant experience than they had expected (Clair, 1987a).

USES OF MUSIC IN THE RECOVERY ROOM

Music used in the recovery room helps patients orient to reality, provides a diversion from the surrounding sounds and activities, and structures time as patients wait for discharge or transfer to a medical unit in the medical center.

During recovery, reality orientation is especially important for patients who have undergone general anesthesia. These patients can be confused and disoriented when they first awaken. Recovery room nurses facilitate patients' reality orientation by calling their names, asking them to move certain body parts such as their toes, and telling them that the procedure is over and that they are in recovery. It takes time to regain consciousness, and patients may be somewhat agitated as they approach consciousness. Patients may attempt to remove or pull at tubes or monitoring equipment lines, or they may attempt to sit up, get out of bed, or strike at nurses who approach them. They may also be alarmed by the automated blood pressure cuff as it inflates and deflates on schedule to measure systolic and diastolic pressures or by the sounds and sensations of other monitoring equipment.

Music may be used to calm the agitation and anxiety of patients in the recovery room by providing them with a predictable, secure environment even before full consciousness is regained. Patients who have experienced music in recovery from general anesthesia have reported that they recognized the sounds they heard as music and that the music was clear and undistorted. Patients who hear music as they awaken from general anesthesia feel a sense of calm and familiarity.

The music that is most effective in calming and orienting patients in the recovery room is music that is familiar to them and music with which they have positive associations. The music is best chosen by the patient before the procedure. Music played in free field for all patients in the recovery room is not recommended, but cannot be avoided for patients who cannot wear headphones (e.g., patients who have surgical dressings on their head, face, or neck). As in the operating room, the best approach for most patients is music played through headphones.

Recovery room nurses have indicated that they found patients much less combative, less confused, and easier to manage when they listened to music than when they did not. They also believed that the patients required less medication to manage their pain (Clair, 1987d). These indications were based on experienced nurses' observations of patients and not on actual measures of patients' medication dosages or behavioral responses. It is possible that the music made the analgesic medications more effective by enhancing relaxation. In fact, the effects of analgesics are increased through relaxation (McCaffery & Pasero, 1999). These patients may have been relaxed by the music because they were calm and quiet as they awakened.

Although there are indications that music played in the recovery room following surgery is viable and effective in increasing patients' comfort and well-being (Macdonald, Mitchell, Dillon, Serpell, Davies, & Ashley, 2003; McCaffery & Locsin, 2004; Thorgaard, Ertman, Hansen, Noerregaard, Hansen, & Spanggaard, 2005), additional research is needed to determine the benefits more clearly. Substantiation of various applications of music through controlled research studies will add information concerning the most effective approaches, the optimum length of time that the music should be played, and the most viable schedule for implementation of music during the recovery process. Until such research has been conducted, people who wish to use music as they recover from anesthesia must decide what music they prefer. Patients scheduled for general anesthesia must consider their waking patterns and their preference for sound or no sound in deciding whether to use music in recovery and in selecting the music they want to hear. Although familiar, preferred music is recommended, it must also be determined whether rousing stimulative music or more gentle sedative music is most appropriate for each individual. Some people awaken quickly with minimal sound stimulation, while others crawl from sleep with maximum sound stimulation. Music selected to suit each patient's normal pattern of waking may best contribute to familiar feelings and well-being, even though return to consciousness following anesthesia is much different from waking from natural sleep.

Should music be used in recovery, the selections must be labeled plainly in order for nursing staff to facilitate their implementation. The sequence of songs must be indicated if more than one selection has been made, and instructions for time of application must be clear.

As patients awaken, they may prefer periodic decreases in volume. In addition, they may develop listening fatigue and may want the music discontinued, at least for a time. It is important for medical staff to check periodically with recovering patients to determine whether the music is still desirable and whether the volume is appropriate.

USES OF MUSIC IN PALLIATIVE CARE

Palliative care focuses on developing and maintaining the best quality of life possible for people who have a disease or condition that is untreatable and incurable. Palliative care incorporates a wide range of interventions that affect physical and emotional comfort and continued social interaction.

Music is a viable approach to maintaining the quality of life of people receiving palliative care for several reasons, including the following:

1. Music provides a basis for reminiscence and life review.

2. Music provides a means for relating to others.

3. Music offers distraction from physical pain and discomfort.

4. Music provides emotional comfort and relief from anxiety.

5. Music provides enjoyment.

6. Music provides release in the last hours of life.

Using Music to Stimulate Reminiscence and Life Review

The literature is replete with articles that describe the importance of reminiscence later in life. Butler (1963) found that reviewing the events and experiences of life was an essential process. Other early research described reminiscence as a way to adapt to change or stress, a source of life validation and self-esteem, a means to evaluate quality of life, and a way to draw upon personal strengths (McMahon & Rhudick, 1964; Merriam & Cross, 1981; Romaniuk & Romaniuk, 1981). Although a number of approaches are used to stimulate memories of life events and experiences, music is an effective facilitator. When people hear certain pieces of music, they naturally recall not only events and experiences, but the feelings associated with them. These musical selections were a part of their lives. Of particular significance were selections whose theme was home life and selections they heard commonly during their young adult years. Wylie (1990) used familiar music with older adults in residential care in order to stimulate discussions of memories. She suggested that music stimulated memories only if it had personal memories associated with it. She recommended that songs that do not stimulate reminiscence should not be used and other selections should be made to stimulate reminiscence. Other clinicians have had positive results using music to prompt memories and reminiscence (Ashida, 2000; Gallagher, Lagman, Walsh, Davis, & LeGrand, 2006; Halstead and Roscoe, 2002; Krout, 2003).

Using Music to Relate to Others

It can be beneficial for people to use music for reminiscence when they are alone, but the benefits increase when they can share their memories with other people. Consequently, in residential care, reminiscing is often done in a group setting. In addition, music can be used during family visits to stimulate memories and discussion about the past. Younger family members may particularly enjoy the stories about the past and may gain a better understanding of their own histories from information concerning their family. Although these discussions can take place without music, mention of a particular song may elicit content that otherwise may have been overlooked.

Participation in music can also provide ways for people to interact nonverbally (Hilliard, 2001). It may provide a context for participation in playing an instrument, dancing, or moving in rhythm with others. Music also provides a context for touching, as when two people dance together. This tactile stimulation is so often missing, especially in the lives of older people. Many times, older people are not touched, except to provide for their physical care needs. Touch is still an important form of stimulation for quality of life for them. Like younger people, older adults need to be held, to have arms wrapped around them, or to have another person sit close, allowing human contact. Although opportunities for physical contact are not generally a part of care plans, they can be incorporated into activities with music. For example, people who can no longer stand or move their feet to dance can still sway to the music with their arms around the shoulders of other people.

Using Music as a Distraction from Physical Pain and Discomfort

People in palliative care are restricted in their options for activity either by their physical conditions or by their inability to function cognitively. It is therefore difficult, if not impossible, for them to implement relaxation approaches either with or without music. Consequently, it is essential that their pain is well managed by medication. Familiar music may provide some additional comfort by eliciting some release of tension. This release may occur when people associate particular selections with nurturing and feelings of well-being. When the release occurs, this music can add to quality of life just by listening to recordings of it; live performances may be even more effective. Relief from pain occurs when a person focuses on music and not on discomfort.

Using Music for Relief from Fear and Anxiety

Music provides relief from fear and anxiety whenever it is familiar and provides comfort through its pleasant associations. Familiar music seems to surround people in comfort and peace. Through music, they have the structure of rhythm and the predictability of melodies, forms, and phrases. People can release their apprehensions as they focus on the familiar, pleasing sounds, which may also have associations of well-being from earlier in their lives.

Using Music for Enjoyment

Sometimes the greatest benefits of music are derived from simply having fun with it. It is essential for people of all ages and abilities to have opportunities for enjoyment, and it is especially true for older people receiving palliative care. Often, their days are filled with people caring for their physical needs and trying to make them comfortable. They may be limited in their physical capacities, which preclude participation in most activities, but they can still enjoy listening to or participating in music when the activity suits their ability level.

Because people enjoy participating in music, whether participation is passive or active, it provides them with a focus for interest and stimulation. The focus relieves boredom and creates opportunities to interact with other people.

Using Music with People in the Final Hours of Life

The music used in the last stage of life, when people are no longer ambulatory and may be moving in and out of consciousness, provides a point of contact between dying people and the people who care for them emotionally and physically (Krout, 2003). For these people, the most appropriate music may be that which was in some way significant to them. Some selections may come from the music families used at holidays, celebrations, and special events and moments in the past. Bringing that music into the present offers an opportunity to reexperience the emotions felt at an earlier time. For loved ones, the music revives and reestablishes the emotional intimacy that may have been missing for some time because of the constraints of illness. Husbands or wives may choose music they danced to with their spouses when they were young, romance was high, and the future was full of hope. The feelings associated with the music can be triggered again, and a review of memories of joyful times can give cause for celebration. Music can range from the music used in courting to music experienced together at later periods of life, provided it is familiar and opens opportunities for people to connect.

Music used in religious rituals can also provide comfort when shared with loved ones, even if they do not seem cognizant or aware of their surroundings. It is possible for music to trigger an awareness response, even if the person is close to death. Awareness responses may include opening the eyes, turning the head toward the source of the music, changing facial expression, crying, or speaking for the first time in several days or weeks. These responses indicate a level of consciousness that families yearn to experience while they wait at the bedside of loved ones who are no longer responsive to their touch or voices.

An illustration of therapeutic music used at the point of death was related by Faith Ullom, a board-certified music therapist who works primarily with older people:

A woman who was in a comatose state and very ill was dying. She had not been responsive for many days, and when her husband visited her, she did not give any indication that she was aware of his presence. I was asked by her family to come and be with them and their loved one in the last moments of the older woman's life. The husband asked me to sing his wife's favorite hymn, "Rock of Ages." I stood behind the family as they gathered around the bed. The man took his wife's hands in his, and as he sat close to her, I began to sing. I had just about finished the last verse when the man began to sob. The heart monitor flat-lined, and it was clear that the woman was dead. I stayed with the family for a few moments, and as I turned to leave, the husband followed me into the hallway. He told me that he had wanted so badly for his wife to let him know that she knew he was with her. He said, "You know, Faith, just before she breathed her last, she gave my hand a little squeeze. She told me 'goodbye.' Thank you for singing. I think it made it possible for her to know we were with her somehow. Anyway, I will always feel like she knew."

Music enabled this family to share emotional closeness with their loved one in the final moments of her life. The music provided them with a way to be with her and to connect with her and one another through a song of which she was particularly fond.

In addition to the emotional closeness music provides to families and loved ones, music has the potential to facilitate release from one state of existence to another through the physical death of the body. Dossey (1994) writes of death as a transition in which the physical body dies, but something fundamental, the soul, remains, and that music thanatology can facilitate the transition between physical and spiritual existence. Music thanatology is a form of palliative care that uses prescriptive music to provide comfort as death occurs (Paxton, 1994). Developed by Therese Schroeder-Sheker, music thanatology follows the traditions developed in medieval Europe that allow people to let go of life at the point of death. Theoretically, the medieval chants that are sung in Latin, which have no beat, time signature, or major and minor tonality, allow people to relax their connection to time and to life. This music is performed live and is adapted to the particular needs of individuals in the spirit of making the last hours of life a part of the life cycle that is beautiful, reverent, dignified, and intimate (Freeman, Caserta, Lund, Rossa, Dowdy, & Partenheimer, 2006; Schroeder-Sheker, 1993). Therefore, music at the point of death is used to create an environment of love and support and to provide comfort to dying people and their families (Paxton, 1994).

CONCLUSION

Music has great potential to bring comfort at times of physical distress associated with surgery, medical procedures, and care provided during illness, disability, and even at the end of life. Common to these times of distress is the lack of control felt by individuals who must experience and endure them. One way to manage the feelings and effects associated with lack of control is to implement techniques that comfort and promote health but that do not interfere in care or treatment processes. Music is integral to such unobtrusive techniques and is compatible with care and treatment procedures. Music is, therefore, viable and efficacious as a therapeutic intervention and may serve to enhance the quality of life for patients in medical care.

REFERENCES

Ashida, S. (2000). The effect of reminiscence music therapy sessions on changes in depressive symptoms in elderly persons with dementia. *Journal of Music Therapy*, 3(3), 170–182.

Biley, F. (1992). Using music in hospital settings. *Nursing Standard*, 6(35), 37–39.

Butler, R. N. (1963). The life review: An interpretation of reminiscence in the aged. *Psychiatry*, 26, 65–76.

Clair, A. A. (1987a). *Discussions with ophthalmic surgical patients: Reaction to music therapy in surgery*. Unpublished observations.

Clair, A. A. (1987b). *Discussions with surgical staff nurses: Reactions to music therapy in surgery*. Unpublished observations.

Clair, A. A. (1987c). *Discussions with transurethral resection of the prostate patients: Reaction to music therapy in surgery*. Unpublished observations.

Clair, A. A. (1987d). *Observation of and discussion with a surgical patient and his recovery nurses*. Unpublished observations.

Clark, M., Isaacks-Downton, G., Wells, N., Redlin-Frazier, S., Eck, C., Hepworth, J. T., & Chakravarthy, B. (2006). Use of preferred music to reduce emotional distress and symptom activity during radiation therapy. *Journal of Music Therapy*, 43(3), 247–265.

Cooke, M., Chaboyer, W., Schluter, P., & Hiratos, M. (2005). The effect of music on preoperative anxiety in day surgery. *Journal of Advanced Nursing*, 52(1), 47–55.

Davis, W., & Gfeller, K. (1999). Music therapy: An historical perspective. In W. Davis, K. Gfeller, & M. Thaut (Eds.), *An introduction to music therapy: Theory and practice* (2nd ed.) (pp. 15–34). Boston: McGraw Hill College.

Deng, G., & Cassileth, B. R. (2005). Integrative oncology: Complementary therapies for pain, anxiety, and mood disturbance. *CA: A Cancer Journal for Clinicians*, 55(2), 109–116.

Dossey, L. (1993). *Healing words: The power of prayer in the practice of medicine*. New York: Harper.

Dossey, L. (1994, August). Medicine's challenge: Recovering the soul. *Messenger*, St. Patrick Hospital Newsletter, Missoula, MT.

Dripps, R. D., Eckenhoff, J. E., & Vandam, L. D. (1988). *Introduction to anesthesia: The principles of safe practice* (7th ed.). Philadelphia: W. B. Saunders.

Freeman, L., Caserta, M., Lund, D., Rossa, S., Dowdy, A., & Partenheimer, A. (2006). Music thanatology: Prescriptive harp music as palliative care for the dying patient. *American Journal of Hospice and Palliative Medicine*, 23(2), 100–104.

Gallagher, L. M., Lagman, R., Walsh, D., Davis, M. P., & LeGrand, S. B. (2006). The clinical effects of music therapy in palliative medicine. *Supportive Care in Cancer*, 14(8), 859–866.

Gaynor, M. L. (2002). *The healing power of sound: Recovery from life-threatening illness using sound, voice, and music*. Boston: Shambhala.

Good, M., Anderson, G. C., Stanton-Hicks, M., Grass, J. A., & Makii, M. (2002). Relaxation and music reduce pain after gynecologic surgery. *Pain Management Nursing*, 3(2), 61–70.

Halstead, M. T., & Roscoe, S. T. (2002). Restoring the spirit at the end of life: Music as an intervention for oncology nurses. *Clinical Journal of Oncology Nurses*, 6(6), 332–336.

Hilliard, R. E. (2001). The use of music therapy in meeting the multidimensional needs of hospice patients and their families. *Journal of Palliative Care*, 17(3), 161–166.

Hodges, D. A. (Ed.). (1996). *Handbook of music psychology* (2nd ed.). St. Louis, MO: MMB Music.

Kenny, D. T., & Faunce, G. (2004). The impact of group singing on mood, coping, and perceived pain in chronic pain patients attending a multidisciplinary pain clinic. *Journal of Music Therapy*, 41(3), 241–258.

Krout, R. E. (2003). Music therapy with imminently dying hospice patients and their families: Facilitating release near time of death. *American Journal of Hospice and Palliative Medicine*, 20(2), 129–134.

Kwekkeboom, K. (2003). Music versus distraction for procedural pain and anxiety in cancer patients. *Oncology Nursing Forum*, 30(3), 433–440.

Lim, P. H., & Locsin, R. (2006). Music as an intervention for pain in five Asian countries. *International Nursing Review*, 53(3), 189–196.

Macdonald, R. A. R., Mitchell, L. A., Dillon, T., Serpell, M. G., Davies, J. B., & Ashley, E. A. (2003). An empirical investigation of the anxiolytic and pain reducing effects of music. *Psychology of Music*, 3(2), 187–203.

Maranto, C. (Ed.). (1991). *Application of music in medicine*. Silver Spring, MD: National Association for Music Therapy.

McCaffery, M., & Pasero, C. (1999). *Pain: Clinical manual* (2nd ed.). St. Louis, MO: Mosby.

McCaffery, R., & Locsin, R. (2004). The effect of music listening on acute confusion and delirium in elders undergoing elective hip and knee surgery. *Journal of Clinical Nursing*, 13(s2), 91–96.

McMahon, A. W., & Rhudick, P. J. (1964). Reminiscing in the aged: An adaptational response. *Archives of General Psychiatry*, 10, 292–298.

Merriam, S., & Cross, L. H. (1981). Aging, reminiscence, and life satisfaction. *Activities, Adaptations and Aging*, 2(1), 39–50.

Patt, R. B., & Kaleka, L. (1990). Recovery from regional anesthesia. In E. Frost (Ed.), *Post anesthesia care unit: Current practices* (2nd ed.) (pp. 106–117). St. Louis, MO: C.V. Mosby.

Paxton, F. (1994). From life to death. *Connecticut College Magazine*, 3(6), 26–29.

Pelletier, C. L. (2004). The effect of music on decreasing arousal due to stress: A meta-analysis. *Journal of Music Therapy*, 41(3), 192–214.

Robb, S. (2000). The effect of therapeutic music interventions on the behavior of hospitalized children in isolation: Developing a contextual support model of music therapy. *Journal of Music Therapy*, 37(2), 118–146.

Robb, S., Nichols, R., Rutan, R., Bishop, B., & Parker, J. (1995). The effects of music assisted relaxation on preoperative anxiety. *Journal of Music Therapy*, 32(1), 2–21.

Romaniuk, M., & Romaniuk, J. F. (1981). Looking back: An analysis of reminiscence functions and triggers. *Experimental Aging Research*, 7(4), 477–489.

Schroeder-Sheker, T. (1993). Music for the dying: A personal account of the new field of music thanatology—History, theories, and clinical narratives. *Advances*, 9(1), 36–48.

Siedliecki, S. L., & Good, M. (2006). Effect of music on power, pain, depression and disability. *Journal of Advanced Nursing*, 54(5), 553–562.

Siegel, B. (1994, November). *The art of healing*. Paper presented at the annual conference of the National Association for Music Therapy, Orlando, FL.

Siegel, B. (1999). *Love, medicine, and miracles* (New ed.). London: Rider & Co.

Standley, J. (1986). Music research in medical/dental treatment: Meta-analysis and clinical applications. *Journal of Music Therapy*, 23(1), 56–122.

Standley, J. (1992). Meta-analysis of research in music and medical treatment: Effect size as a basis for comparison across multiple dependent and independent variables. In R. Spintge & R. Droh (Eds.), *Music medicine* (pp. 364–378). St. Louis, MO: MMB Music.

Standley, J. (1996). Music research in medical/dental treatment: An update of a prior meta-analysis. In C. Furman (Ed.), *Effectiveness of music therapy procedures: Documentation of research and clinical practice* (2nd ed.) (pp. 1–60). Silver Spring, MD: National Association for Music Therapy.

Standley, J. M. (2000). Music research in medical treatment. In AMTA (Ed.), *Effectiveness of music therapy procedures: Documentation of research and clinical practice* (3rd ed.) (pp. 1–64). Silver Spring, MD: American Music Therapy Association.

Taylor, D. (1981). Music in general hospital treatment from 1900 to 1950. *Journal of Music Therapy*, 18(2), 62–73.

Thaut, M. H. (2005). Physiological and motor responses to music stimuli. In R. Unkefer & M. H. Thaut (Eds.), *Music therapy in the treatment of adults with mental disorders* (pp. 33–41). Gilsum, NH: Barcelona.

Thorgaard, P., Ertmann, E., Hansen, V., Noerregaard, A., Hansen, V., & Spanggaard, L. (2005). Designed sound and music environment in postanaesthesia care units—A multicentre study of patients and staff. *Intensive and Critical Care Nursing*, 21(4), 220–225.

Whitehead-Pleaux, A. M. (2006). The effects of music therapy on pediatric patients' pain and anxiety during donor site dressing change. *Journal of Music Therapy*, 43(2), 136–153.

Wylie, M. E. (1990). A comparison of the effects of old familiar songs, antique objects, historical summaries, and general questions on the reminiscence of nursing home residents. *Journal of Music Therapy*, 27(1), 2–12.

Chapter 8

Music in Physical Rehabilitation

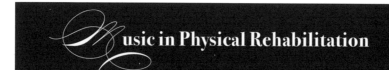

usic in Physical Rehabilitation

Beyond age 70, the potential for physiological changes that lead to multiple medical and social problems increases every year (Edelberg, 2004). These changes affect the ability of a person to perform self-care activities that are a part of a desirable quality of life. When serious physiological changes occur, physical rehabilitation is required to restore physical function to the premorbid level (if possible) and to prevent functional decline (Studenski & Woods Duncan, 2004). Rehabilitation is so essential to health and well-being that few people should be excluded from rehabilitation programs, even when they have little chance of regaining full function (Holohan-Bell & Brummel-Smith, 1999). The potential for regaining full function is determined by many factors, including premorbid condition, prognosis for recovery, and environmental resources. These factors must be assessed so that an appropriate rehabilitation program can be designed and implemented. The primary concern in any rehabilitation program is whether the individual possesses sufficient self-care abilities to live alone, has self-care deficits that require assistance at home, or has self-care deficits that are so pronounced that residential care is necessary. Self-care abilities vary greatly, beginning with advanced activities of daily living (ADLs), which represent voluntary physical and social functions, such as activities associated with employment, recreational exercise, gardening, travel, participation in religious groups, and involvement in social clubs (Reuben, Laliberte, Hiris, & Mor, 1990). The ability to function in these activities may diminish over a person's lifetime, but the activities are not essential to maintaining independence. Intermediate ADLs determine whether a person can continue to live alone independently and include abilities such as managing financially, remaining mobile, and maintaining daily activities. The most basic level of intermediate ADLs includes abilities associated with personal care (e.g., bathing, eating, and toileting). Individuals who require assistance with basic ADLs need a great deal of daily care; if their abilities become sufficiently limited, they may require 24-hour residential nursing care.

Although the benefits of rehabilitation programs are widely acknowledged, participation in these programs is not easily accepted by all people who could benefit from them. This is for several reasons. First, people with physical abilities that restrict range of motion find exercise painful. Bearing one's weight can become uncomfortable and has the potential to discourage any movement; thus, locomotion may become so slow that it is more convenient to use a wheelchair. Second, some people who believe that bed rest is optimal for any physical ailment resist suggestions to incorporate movement and exercise as essential components into their rehabilitation. Third, people with losses in physical functioning may slip into a depression so severe that they avoid all activity, especially uncomfortable activity. Generally, rehabilitation can be difficult, even for people who are committed to participating in rehabilitation. Although they wish to function well and to preserve their options for living independently, they welcome occasional relief from the physical and emotional discomfort and from rehabilitation itself.

CARDIOVASCULAR REHABILITATION

Cardiovascular disease is the leading cause of death in the United States. Approximately one in three American adults have one or more types of cardiovascular disease, of which nearly half are 65 and older (American Heart Association, 2008). Inactivity is one of the primary causes of cardiovascular disease, and aerobic exercise is an essential component of its therapy, even for people with myocardial infarction (American Heart Association, 2008). Despite the positive results associated with rehabilitative exercise, maintaining adherence to the rehabilitation program is a major problem. Only 10–20% of eligible individuals participate in cardiac rehabilitation (Rozanski & Blumenthal, 2006), and at least 50% of the individuals referred for cardiac rehabilitation drop out of the program (Digenio et al., 1991; Dishman, 1982). This attrition is the result of intolerance of or maladaptation to the discomfort experienced during exercise. Therefore, there are indications that distraction from the physical work of exercise could encourage adherence to cardiac rehabilitation programs.

Using Music in Cardiac Rehabilitation

Participation in and adherence to any rehabilitation program must be monitored carefully by medical staff. Medical practitioners are generally open to anything that will promote participation and adherence to the program. Often, music is integral to promoting adher-

ence. Music should be incorporated carefully into a cardiac rehabilitation program under the following conditions. First, it is essential to
have approval from the physician of record before introducing music
into a rehabilitation program, provided it is not already included.

Second, the effects of any music that is used must be monitored carefully. If the music causes a negative change in mood or if it
seems burdensome, it should be changed. The only way to influence
a person's mood with music is to try particular selections until the desired effect is achieved. The effect of the music is usually determined
quickly, so if positive responses are not achieved soon after the music
is introduced, other music should be selected. No single type of music
triggers the same response in all people (i.e., music that improves the
mood of one person may not improve the mood of another person).

Third, participants' physical reactions to music should be
monitored. Music may be so successful as a distraction that people
are not aware of their physical responses to exercise. Signs of fatigue
or overexertion may be ignored if the music is too distracting. The
possibility of injury exists for people who become so involved in their
selected music that they may fall asleep or become less attentive, particularly while exercising on exercise machinery. To prevent sleep or
lack of awareness, the volume of the music should be lowered so participants can more capably monitor their posture and activity.

Fourth, in order for the music to be effective, the tempo of
the music must be matched to the tempo of the exercise movements.
As recovery progresses and faster speeds can be incorporated into the
exercises, the music should be changed to match these speeds.

Fifth, the combination of music and meditation is powerful;
thus, guided imagery sessions must be led only by those with professional training. People who may have attended a music and imagery
presentation at a conference or received an introduction to music and
imagery by reading magazines or books may be tempted to experiment. However, such experimentation may result in harmful responses in participants, particularly if they experience flashbacks of painful
memories and the unresolved feelings associated with them. Other
participants may be particularly vulnerable to suggested images that
may evoke distressing associations. (See Chapter 5 for an explanation
of the training program Guided Imagery and Music.)

Finally, incorporating music into an exercise program may

not be suitable for everyone. Although rare, there are people who do not particularly enjoy music and prefer not to have it be part of their environment.

Like many other exercise programs, cardiac exercise programs are organized into four stages: warm-up stretches, active participation, cool-down, and relaxation/meditation. A typical cardiac rehabilitation program requires participation in exercise a minimum of three times per week, consisting of warm-up stretches, either walking or riding a stationary bicycle, cool-down stretches, and relaxation/meditation. Warm-up stretches may be performed in a group with music played in free field. (Preferences of the participants should be surveyed to ensure that they all approve the musical selections before beginning the exercise.) The group setting allows rehabilitation therapists to provide instructions for all participants and additionally provides an opportunity for participants to work with other people in recovery and rehabilitation following a heart attack.

The active participation stage of the program eliminates the music played in free field. Participants exercise individually, wearing small portable players with headsets. Each participant selects his or her preferred music, and the music is monitored to ensure that its tempo is suitable to the exercise. All participants are encouraged to proceed at their own pace, while medical personnel monitor their heart rate and blood pressure.

The participants reassemble in a group to perform cool-down stretches and relaxation/meditation. Music, agreed upon by the group before these segments of the program, plays in free field and the medical staff leads participants in the appropriate activities.

MacNay (1995) examined the effects of music used during rehabilitative exercises in case studies of four cardiac patients at a U.S. Department of Veterans Affairs medical center in the Midwest. MacNay theorized that using the subjects' preferred music during exercise would provide a cue, or distraction, that would decrease their perceptions of exertion, would improve their mood, and decrease the estimated time needed for the exercise. The results of his study showed that the subjects thought their mood improved with music during exercise and that they estimated that the duration of exercise was shorter with music than without it. However, the results did not indicate that subjects thought the exercise required less exertion with music than without.

One of MacNay's subjects was a veteran who had received shrapnel injuries to his legs that caused pain when he walked or exercised his legs. This subject had been sedentary up until his heart attack and his subsequent involvement in the cardiac rehabilitation program. He reported that the exercise was difficult and painful, but he knew that it was necessary for his survival. He agreed to participate in an exercise program using music he preferred, although he expressed reservations as to its effectiveness. To the veteran's surprise, the music distracted him from his pain and made completing the exercises possible. In a follow-up interview 6 months later, the man was still exercising regularly with music. He said that because he had adhered to the program, he was able to mow his lawn, something he could not accomplish on his own before his heart attack. Although he needed to sit and rest his legs periodically, he was pleased that he no longer had to hire someone to mow the lawn. He boasted that he was in as good shape as he was when he received his honorable military discharge.

MacNay concluded from his small sample study that music may exert a positive influence on the perceptions of cardiac patients during exercise. He postulated that if listening to music decreases perceived exertion, improves mood, and decreases estimates of time needed for exercise, individuals (including older adults) can participate in vital exercise programs with fewer complaints of fatigue, better moods, and for a longer time. Recent studies examining the impact of music in the exercise regimens and treatment plans of individuals in cardiac healthcare support MacNay's initial findings (Hanser & Mandel, 2005; Mandel, 1996; Metzger, 2004; Murrock, 2002).

STROKE REHABILITATION

Of all strokes, about 71% occur in people over age 65. Approximately 88% of stroke deaths occur in individuals aged 65 and older (American Heart Association, 2008). Treatment for a stroke is provided in three phases, as follows:

1. The acute phase, in which abilities and deficits are determined and attention is focused on cognitive processing, emotional responses, motor function, postural control, sensory perception, speech, and

language

2. The subacute phase, in which efforts are made to prevent further deterioration from complications of stroke

3. The chronic phase, in which the goal of treatment is to maintain functional levels, although residual neurological deficits impair independent functioning.

Individuals in the chronic phase must cope with the depression associated with their deficits, adjust to living at home or in a nursing home with adaptive equipment, compensate for changing roles and responsibilities, and rely on family and other support systems (Studenski & Woods Duncan, 2004). The chronic phase presents both physical and emotional challenges to both the people who have had a stroke and their caregivers.

Using Music in Stroke Rehabilitation

Generally, rehabilitation begins as soon as the person who has had a stroke is medically stable. The rehabilitation process is slow and involves a broad spectrum of disciplines. Therapeutic applications of music across this spectrum can include music that provides a familiar, comforting environment within the medical setting, music integrated into speech-language therapy, music integrated into physical therapy to develop muscle tone and eventual ambulation training, and music to restore socialization and emotional well-being.

Music may initially be used to provide comfort, but it must be used discriminately because any sensory stimulation may cause severe discomfort. In fact, some patients cannot cope with any sound at all, including music, until after the initial hours following the stroke. Music familiar to the person who has had a stroke can provide feelings of security and predictability in the hospital. Some individuals have reported that music was the first thing they recognized and felt a sense of comfort about as they awakened from coma produced by the stroke. The music must be played at low volume and intermittently. If played continuously, the music will be disregarded and its potential to elicit positive responses will be lost. It can be used at times of wakefulness and particularly at times of agitation.

Not all people are comforted by the same types of music. When the person who has had a stroke cannot communicate, family, spouses, or friends should be consulted to help determine the most efficacious music. If this information is unknown or not available, music selections can be tried until a relaxation response is evident.

Using Music in Speech Rehabilitation

Often, speech impairments are the result of the brain damage caused by a stroke. Speech impairments can take the following forms (*Dorland's Illustrated Medical Dictionary*, 2000): apraxia, a loss of ability to carry out familiar, purposeful movement without the presence of paralysis or other motor or sensory impairment; dysarthria, the imperfect articulation of speech because of muscular control disturbances resulting from damage to the central or peripheral nervous system; aphasia, a defect or loss of expression because of brain injury or disease that results in distorted speech, writing, or singing, or in a disturbance in spoken or written language comprehension. Aphasia can occur in many forms, and the forms can be combined in some individuals.

Although patients may be comatose, paralyzed, or otherwise unresponsive, they may be aware on some level of what is said in their presence. No one knows with exact certainty what is understood by severely injured people when discussions are held in their presence. If spoken words have no cognitive meaning for them, the emotions in the speaker's voice may communicate a wide range of messages, from hope and encouragement to dejection and despair. Visitors should be cautioned to speak as though every word is understood clearly by the patient, even if he or she is comatose or completely paralyzed, as in the following vignette:

> When Mrs. Wilan recovered her speech many weeks after her stroke, she spoke angrily about the conversations that took place at her bedside during the early stage of her illness. She said that her family and friends held conversations in the room as if she was not present. Although she could not open her eyes or respond in any way, she heard and understood every word. Her own fears and anxieties with the sudden onset of her disability were magnified by these conversations—talk

of how she may never recover, how she could be a vegetable for the rest of her life—and she fell into a deep depression. Mrs. Wilan said that she was furious that she was forced to battle not only her own physical helplessness but the extreme discouragement brought on by conversations that occurred, as she put it, "as though I was a piece of furniture, a lifeless form lying on the bed who could comprehend nothing!" She was very angry that these conversations increased her distress at a time when she needed support, hopefulness, and encouragement.

Singing to Promote Speech Rehabilitation. Singing has long helped rehabilitate people with neurological impairments. Research results, such as those of Cohen (1992), indicate positive outcomes. These results have come out of the use of various approaches, including melodic intonation therapy, in which singing is used either to enhance speech or to increase speech production (Albert, Sparks, & Helm, 1973; Baker, 2000; Blumstein & Cooper, 1974; Bonakdarpour, Eftekharzadeh, & Ashayeri, 2000; Krauss & Galloway, 1982; Laughlin, Naeser, & Gordon, 1979; Sparks, Helm, & Albert, 1974; Sparks & Holland, 1976; Wilson, Parsons, & Reutens, 2006).

Cohen (1992) examined the effects of singing instruction on the production of speech of people with neurological impairments. She was interested in improving the fundamental frequency (tone of voice), the fundamental frequency variability (changes in tone of voice), the vocal intensity, the rate of speech, and the verbal intelligibility. A total of 8 individuals were studied, 2 controls and 6 experimental subjects. The 6 subjects, who were residents at two rehabilitation facilities, participated in singing treatment sessions for 30 minutes 3 times per week for 3 weeks. The controls did not participate in the sessions. Before the series of singing treatment sessions began and after the final session, the speech of all 8 subjects was recorded on tape as they described the content of two pictures. The sessions for the experimental subjects began with 5 minutes of physical exercise, which involved moving the face, neck, head, shoulders, and upper torso while calming music played. Cohen followed these exercises with 10 minutes of vocal warm-ups, comprising both breathing and vocal exercises, and 5 minutes of rhythmic speech drills, which consisted of chanting famous sayings or song lyrics. The sessions concluded with 10 minutes of singing songs subjects knew well before the stroke.

Experts rated the pre- and posttest audiotapes for both experimental (N = 6) and control subjects (N = 2). Their conclusions showed that experimental subjects who attended between seven and nine sessions achieved better results than subjects who attended fewer sessions. Trends in both directions were observed for all subjects, as follows:

1. Of the original 6 experimental subjects, 4 decreased in their fundamental frequency, whereas 2 increased in their fundamental frequency.

2. Both control subjects decreased their fundamental frequency from pre- to posttest.

3. Of the 6 experimental subjects, 4 increased their fundamental frequency variability, which indicated their ability to vary the way they expressed themselves.

4. Neither control subject experienced improvement in variability.

5. Intensity increased in the voices of 2 experimental subjects. Consequently, singing seemed to help them speak louder.

6. Between the pre- and the posttests, 4 experimental subjects improved their rates of speech.

Cohen concluded that singing has the potential to help rehabilitate the speech of people with neurological impairments, including people with apraxia, dysarthria, and Broca's (expressive) aphasia. She recommended further study with larger subject samples that include control subjects. She also recommended making comparisons between group and individual sessions and among different types of vocal participation, including singing and rhythmic chanting. In addition, she noted that the etiology of neurological impairments, the degree of damage, medications, age, and other variables were influences on the study results.

Cohen and Masse (1993) conducted a study of 32 people with neurological impairments to determine the effects of rhythmic chanting instruction (N = 9), singing instruction (N = 9), and no instruction (control) (N = 14) on the rate and verbal intelligibility of speech. The subjects were each assigned randomly to one type of instruction. A comparison of pre- and posttest assessment data gathered over 9 weeks yielded increased rates of 21 words per minute for the rhythmic chanting group, 23 words per minute for the singing group, and a decrease of 2 words per minute for the control group. Subjects who sang experienced greater improvement in the rate and verbal intelligibility of speech than subjects who chanted rhythms, and subjects in both treatments improved more than control subjects. In addition, verbal intelligibility scores increased by 21% for the singing group, whereas both rhythm and control groups decreased in verbal intelligibility by 5%. These results were influenced by age. That is, because older subjects tended to be impaired as a result of stroke and cerebral palsy, they were more likely to improve than younger subjects who were diagnosed with progressive neurological conditions.

Cohen and Masse noted that subjects in either the singing or the rhythm group experienced increases in vocal intensity and that subjects in the singing group also increased their vocal range. Both vocal intensity and vocal range are essential to speech and language, and Cohen and Masse recommend the inclusion of these elements in future studies.

Some persons who have experienced a severe stroke have dysphagia, or the inability to swallow food or fluids, which seriously affects life quality and can threaten survival when a blocked airway and/or aspiration pneumonia occurs (Perry, 2001). The process of moving food or liquid from the mouth into the stomach while preventing aspiration into the respiratory tract is very complex (Broussard & Altschuler, 2000), and damage to any part of the system results in a swallowing disorder (Logemann, 1995). Treatment is usually provided by speech-language pathologists who implement a set of exercises designed to progressively improve swallowing function, including those that strengthen the laryngeal closure, a critical mechanism for airway protection during swallowing (Mendelsohn & Martin, 1993). Adherence to the exercise program is often poor and persons therefore fail to develop the best outcomes possible (C. Lett, personal communication, October 25, 2005). For those who participate in an exercise regimen to strengthen swallowing, there is a risk of cardiac death and cardiac arrhythmias resulting from prolonged voluntary closure of the glottis (Chaudhuri, Hildner, Brady, Hutchins, Aliga, & Abadilla, 2002). Therefore there is a need for an exercise program that facilitates engagement while managing cardiac risks.

To test the potential of music therapy enhancement for swallowing treatment, Kim (2006) designed a singing protocol to entrain breathing and to strengthen the voluntary and involuntary movements of the tongue, lips, jaws, and larynx. She based her protocol design upon the concept of entrainment supported by laboratory research conducted by Thaut (1999) and associates and upon Oral Motor and Respiratory Exercises (OMREX), a technique that facilitates speech and respiratory functions through musical components of vocalization, singing, chanting, or playing instruments (Thaut, 1999). Kim's protocol incorporated music as a cueing mechanism to support the physical functions involved in speech, breathing, and swallowing.

In a preliminary test of her protocol, Kim delivered treatment to six persons who had severe dysphagia due to stroke. Results after six sessions revealed statistically significant improvements in laryngeal function and further statistically significant improvements after the 12th session, including decreased drool, deeper and more controlled respirations, and appropriate speech pitch, among other improved speech characteristics. Kim concluded persons' physiological mechanisms for swallowing were restored by providing auditory timing cues and facilitating voice production through singing that replicated the muscle movements involved in the swallowing process. Kim will continue to test her protocol with larger numbers of persons to provide evidence for whether (1) persons have better responses to musical cues than spoken cues especially for those who have disturbances in thinking or memory, (2) improvements happen more quickly with a singing protocol as compared with traditional speech therapy, and (3) individual accommodations provided through musical cues facilitate adherence and participation effort to boost speech therapy outcomes.

Using Music in Physical Rehabilitation

A study conducted by a music therapist in consultation with an occupational therapist showed the effectiveness of music in motivating people to participate in the rehabilitation of their hand grasp on the affected side following stroke (Confrancesco, 1985). In this study, three patients who had been in physical rehabilitation for at least 5 weeks participated as subjects. Their hand grasp strength was assessed using a Jamar Adjustable Dynamometer before and after each music therapy treatment session. Subjects were also required to participate in a test before any music therapy treatment was introduced and a test after all treatment sessions. The tests included a 9-hole peg test, a 15-hole peg test, a test to stack graduated boxes, assessments of coordination and functional tasks, and assessments of music-related expression and behavior. Treatment was implemented in five 30- to 35-minute sessions each week for 3 weeks. Treatments initially included playing a tambourine by holding it in the right hand and hitting it with the affected left hand, holding drumsticks in a hook grasp while playing a drum and cymbal, and holding a clave (small cylindrical wooden sticks that are held in cupped hands and struck together) in each hand and hitting them together in a variety of rhythmic patterns. Once these skills were mastered, subsequent sessions included moving fingers individually, using the piano keyboard to increase dexterity; playing the autoharp, using a pick in the left hand and pressing the chord buttons with the right hand; and playing tom-toms, holding a drumstick in each hand and alternating right and left drum strikes. These applications enhanced hand-eye motor coordination skills, individual finger movements, and lateral prehension (grasping with the hands). Each treatment session ended with relaxation training.

Results of the study showed music therapy treatment improved bilateral movement, functional skills, and coordination. Although motor gains on the left side of the body were not as substantial as those on the right side resulting from damage to the right hemisphere of the brain, the music therapy sessions affected motor function markedly. In addition, subjects improved in measures of expression.

The implications of this study are that people who participate in physical rehabilitation using music are likely to benefit, even after a short period of time. It may be that the music entices them to participate and motivates them to adhere to the program.

The rehabilitation program for restoration of motor function following stroke is long and arduous. At first, an individual who has had a stroke may lack the ability to initiate movement and may also lack the range of motion necessary to assume postures. Extensive physical rehabilitation is required to bring the person through the developmental motor sequence until ambulation and gait training is possible (Kisner & Colby, 2007). Throughout this process, people may benefit from the motor organization provided by rhythmic aural stimulation. Research has demonstrated that sounds, particularly music, excite responses in two ways: signals are sent from the cochlea (the organ of hearing) simultaneously to the cerebral cortex for processing in the brain, and to the spinal cord, where they excite motor neurons that in turn stimulate muscular response. The reaction time to sounds is brief (Pal'tsev & El'ner, 1967; Rossignol & Melville Jones, 1976). Thus, repetitive rhythmic auditory stimuli can synchronize with motor neural activity during a rhythmic motor task (e.g., hopping) and provide motor organization and patterns of response (Rossignol & Melville Jones, 1976).

Thaut (1988) described motor activity as a series of repeated acts that occur through time and described rhythm as repeated events that also occur through time. He determined that motor activity is related to rhythm in that they both have the components of consistent repetition and organization through time. Thaut drew this conclusion from his review of research reports that indicate that people have the ability to perceive and discriminate rhythmic stimuli and that the synchronization of motor rhythm patterns is dependent on individuals' training, experience with movement, and exposure to rhythmic stimuli. Rhythmic stimuli can take many forms, but the most consistently efficient form is rhythmic auditory cueing (Cooper & Glassow, 1982; Huff, 1972; Lhamon & Goldstone, 1974; Luft et al., 2004; Rochester et al., 2005; Rubenstein, Giladi, & Hausdorff, 2002; Thomas & Moon, 1976).

When the motor abilities that contribute to physical independence and quality of life have been damaged through disease or injury (e.g., stroke), people need to relearn these abilities. Observations of the effects of music and rhythmic pulse on gait in people who had experienced strokes demonstrated that subjects showed some improvement (Clair & O'Konski, 2006; Prassas, Thaut, McIntosh, & Rice, 1997; Staum, 1983; Thaut, McIntosh, & Rice, 1997). Thaut and colleagues have since made great inroads in the consideration of the effects of rhythmic auditory cueing on ambulation gait in rehabilitating people who have had strokes. Thaut, McIntosh, Prassas, and Rice (1992b) studied the effect of rhythmic auditory cueing on the gait patterns of people without disabilities. They measured three walking cadences in 16 subjects to determine the timing of the stride cycle (heel strike, mid-stance, push off, acceleration of the swing leg) and the timing and amplitude of electromyographic activity in normal gait. Walking was accompanied by a music stimulus that consisted of an original Renaissance-style piece composed on a synthesizer in 4/4 time that was played in woodwind, harpsichord, and percussion timbres. Superimposed on the 4/4 time were accented first and third beats, which enhanced the rhythm.

Each subject was asked to walk at three different tempos. The first was his or her preferred tempo. Then the rhythmic music stimulus was matched to the preferred tempo and subjects walked while the music played. The second tempo was slightly slower than the subjects' preferred tempo. They were to walk without music and then the rhythmic stimulus was matched to this tempo while they walked. The third tempo was slightly faster than the subjects' preferred tempo. Again, they were instructed to walk without music and then the rhythmic stimulus was added to match the cadence.

Results showed a significant difference in stride arrhythmia between the rhythm and the nonrhythmic conditions, with the average stride time decreasing from an average of 16.9 milliseconds without rhythm to an average of 12.8 milliseconds with rhythm. The stride deviations became smaller with rhythmic auditory cueing, and the researchers concluded that the external auditory rhythm caused the gait to become more symmetrical. In addition, electromyographic analysis showed a decreased variability in electromyographic activity and more focused electromyographic patterns when rhythmic auditory cueing was used in the preferred and the slower walking tempos. Thaut and colleagues concluded that the electromyographic readings indicated a change in neural activity with rhythmic music and that rhythmic auditory cueing generally caused the gait to become more efficient, even though subjects had normal motor functions.

Using the same rhythmic stimulus, Thaut, McIntosh, Prassas, and Rice (1992a) studied the effects of rhythmic auditory cueing on gait in people without disabilities ($N = 8$) and in people who had strokes ($N = 2$), cerebellar disorder ($N = 1$), and transverse myelitis ($N = 1$). Subjects were asked to repeat the gait patterns of the earlier study. Gastrocnemius (calf) muscle electromyography, stride cycle time, and videotaped kinematics were analyzed. The electromyographics of people who had neurological disorders were similar to those of people without such disorders. The subjects' electromyographic profiles showed later onsets, shorter durations, and more focused amplitude ratios during leg stance with rhythm than without it. In addition, temporal strides showed less deviation between the legs with rhythm than without it. People with abnormal gaits showed marked improvements with rhythmic auditory cueing. The researchers concluded that rhythmic auditory cueing made walking more efficient in both people without and people with neurological disabilities. They postulated that this efficiency is the result of alterations in neural activity with auditory rhythm, in which more neurons in the lower neuron pool are stimulated into action for a more focused and consistent muscular response.

Thaut and McIntosh (1992) studied rhythmic auditory cueing in an expanded subject pool that included 16 unimpaired subjects and 10 subjects who had suffered strokes. The subjects walked without and then with rhythmic auditory cueing. The results of the study showed statistically significant changes for all subjects in improved stride rhythmicity, decreased deviations in electromyographic onset and durations for gastrocnemius and anteriortibialis (muscle on the front of the long bone below the knee) muscles, delayed and shortened gastrocnemius activation, and increased integrated amplitude ratios for gastrocnemius activity. These changes indicate more efficient gait and better motor control. The researchers concluded that rhythmic auditory cueing was effective as a neuromuscular rehabilitation technique.

A study by Thaut, McIntosh, Prassas, and Rice (1993) reported the effects of rhythmic auditory cueing on the hemiparetic gait of people who had strokes. Again, the results were marked improvement during the rhythmic auditory cueing. The weight-bearing stance time for the paretic (slight paralysis) side improved with rhythm, which made the stride more symmetrical. In addition, muscle activation on the paretic side improved, and electromyographic variability between the two sides decreased when rhythmic auditory cueing was added. The researchers concluded that there was a strong connection between motor activation and the rhythmic auditory cueing that provided subjects with gait control.

Using rhythmic auditory cueing in gait rehabilitation with 20 subjects who had strokes, Thaut (1994) required subjects to walk without and then with rhythmic auditory cueing matched to the gait cadence. Subjects were assigned either to a control group that participated in conventional gait training or to an experimental group that participated in conventional gait training augmented with rhythmic auditory cueing. All subjects were pre- and posttested without rhythmic auditory cueing. Results of stride, surface electromyography, and videography analyses showed significant increases in gait velocity and symmetry and reductions in double limb support (subjects could alternate feet without stepping feet together, as one might do when using crutches) for subjects who received rhythmic auditory cueing along with conventional gait training. Thus, rhythmic auditory cueing was successful in rehabilitating the hemiparetic gait of the subjects who had stroke.

Although the work of Thaut and colleagues is complex and involves sophisticated measurement protocols, the outcomes are clear: rhythmic auditory cues presented during gait training cause walking to become more symmetrical, more efficient, and better balanced in people who have lost the ability to ambulate as a result of stroke. Videos of subjects with strokes walking with and without music show marked differences and demonstrate the immediate, positive effect of rhythmic auditory cueing on the ability to ambulate. The results of these studies are exciting and show great potential for application in physical rehabilitation programs for, as well as provide hope and encouragement to, people who have had strokes.

A recent clinical application of rhythmic auditory stimulation (RAS) in a hospital rehabilitation setting tested effectiveness on a number of evidence-based, clinical outcomes (Hayden, Clair, Johnson, & Otto, 2007). These included the (1) One-limb Stance, a measure of postural stability in young and elderly adults (Goldie, Evans, & Bach, 1992; Seiger & Hirschfeld, 2004); (2) characteristic gait measures of cadence, velocity, and stride length; (3) the Timed Up and Go Test, a test used to predict the probability for falls while hospitalized for stroke rehabilitation (Andersson, Kamwendo, Seiger, & Appelros, 2006); (4) the functional reach test, which is used to assess balance impairments and changes in balance over time (Duncan, Weiner, Chandler, & Studenski, 1990); (5) the degree of forward head tilt, which correlates with further risk for stroke (Tsunoda, Aikawa, Murakami, Sakai, & Kikkawa, 2003; Tsunoda et al., 2005); and (6) the Ysavage Geriatric Depression Screening Scale.

This clinical study of 15 patients in acute rehabilitation for gait training was conducted in a wait-list control design where 5 patients received RAS enhanced gait training for 30 sessions, 5 patients waited until the 10th of 30 sessions to begin the RAS enhanced gait training, and 5 waited until the 20th of 30 sessions to have RAS enhanced gait training. Measurement outcomes improved statistically significantly over time for one-limb stance, cadence, velocity, stride length, and posture head tilt, no matter how long participants waited to have RAS. There were no statistically significant changes in the Timed Up and Go Test, the Functional Reach Test, and the Ysavage Geriatric Depression Screening Scale.

When changes in outcomes were examined according to the point at which RAS was introduced into the gait training, statistically significant improvements were made in the one-limb stance by those who received RAS for all 30 sessions when compared to those who waited for 20 sessions and received it for the last 10 sessions. Cadence improved statistically significantly more with early implementation of RAS into the treatment program.

This study hints that early introduction of RAS into gait training improves clinical outcomes for one-limb stance and cadence. Further testing with larger numbers of participants is required to confirm these results. The study clearly demonstrated that the clinical protocol developed for the incorporation of RAS into traditional gait training is easy to administer, requires no additional time for implementation, is not obtrusive, and is practical to integrate into physical therapy sessions.

Using Music to Restore Socialization and Emotional Well-Being

People who have had strokes need to grieve. Initially, their grief is compounded by fears and anxieties about their condition. These feelings may be compounded further by an inability to express feelings verbally. Consequently, social contact with loved ones is lost. The frustration that results from the inability to communicate and to express emotions associated with their debilitation can lead to depression and a lack of motivation to participate in rehabilitation.

Singing to Promote Socialization and Emotional Expression. Music, especially singing, can provide an outlet for the communication of thoughts and feelings to loved ones after a stroke. The following vignette shows how singing helped a woman whose speech was impaired by a stroke to communicate with her family.

> After her stroke, Mrs. King could not speak. Her adult children visited her in the rehabilitation hospital every day and talked to her throughout their visits. She could respond to them only by crying. Mrs. King's children found their visits with their mother heartbreaking and tried everything they could to make her happy and end the crying. They washed and styled her hair, manicured her fingernails, and brought pictures from home to show her the traditional family decorations they had installed for the holiday season. Mrs. King continued to respond by crying.

> Mrs. King's roommate, Mrs. Norbert, received a visit from a friend, Ms. O'Connor, who was a music therapist. Ms. O'Connor asked Mrs. Norbert about Mrs. King. Mrs. Norbert encouraged her friend to speak informally with Mrs. King's family.

> Ms. O'Connor spoke with Mrs. King's family, inquiring about her possible response to singing. The family indicated that Mrs. King loved to sing, but that she sang only in church. After inquiring about Mrs. King's favorite hymns, Ms. O'Connor suggested that the family sing them to her. The family was told that it was possible that Mrs. King would join in the singing, but that even if she could not sing along, it was likely she would be comforted by the music and her family. It would also help structure the time during their visits.

> That afternoon the family began singing to Mrs. King, and to everyone's surprise, she joined in. Mrs. King was astonished

that she could sing along with her children, and this made her laugh so hard that at times she could barely sing. It was difficult to determine whether her inability to sing some of the words was the result of her stroke or her joyous laughter.

In a subsequent visit to Mrs. Norbert, Ms. O'Connor learned that Mrs. King's children were singing with their mother every day. Mrs. Norbert confided, "There's so much racket going on every afternoon, I can't hear my soap operas!" However, she said she was glad that Mrs. King seemed so much better.

Mrs. King still faced hours of speech-language pathology and occupational and physical therapy to relearn the skills that would make it possible for her to return home. However, she was motivated to participate in rehabilitation because of the success she experienced in singing her much-loved music with her children. Her success also provided reassurance and joy to her children, who needed to feel that they were helping their mother rather than making her cry.

It may be possible for members of other families to communicate with loved ones who have had strokes by singing to them. Before doing so, family members should consult the attending physician. Some families may need to refrain from immediately stimulating an individual who has recently had a stroke and for whom stimulation is contraindicated. The attending physician will indicate when sensory stimulation can begin. The physician will also caution families not to set their expectations too high. The area and extent of the damage caused by stroke may clarify what type of and when vocal response can be expected. It may be that the stroke has impaired the ability to sing or it may take time for the person to respond.

Some family members or other visitors may be reluctant to sing. Often the suggestion to do so is met with objections such as "I have a terrible voice" or "I can't carry a tune." Their lack of confidence can be overcome through their commitment to their loved ones' treatment and recovery. It is essential that these people know that it is not their vocal quality that is important to the loved one but the sound of their familiar voice. Pressure should never be placed on people to sing along with others if they do not wish to sing, but to do so when alone with a loved one without interruption may provide a nonthreatening way to begin.

Playing Instrumental Music to Promote Socialization and Emotional Expression. Therapeutic applications of music during and after rehabilitation from stroke may include playing various musical instruments (Jeong & Kim, 2007). Instruments that will provide immediate successful experiences must be selected, and certain adaptations of the instruments may be required in order for people to manipulate them. Consultation with a qualified music therapist can ensure the most appropriate instrument selection and approach.

Often, percussion instruments help provide motivation for engaging in bilateral upper body activity, which can promote range of motion and can provide an outlet for all types of emotional expression, as in the following vignette:

> Mr. Garcia was in rehabilitation for gait training following a lower limb amputation. When Ms. Reno, the music therapist, approached him in his room, Mr. Garcia was quiet and withdrawn. He was alone, so she asked if he would like to play a drum she had with her. He refused, saying he did not feel like playing anything. Ms. Reno sat and spoke with him about the kind of music he liked. He mumbled that he liked Duke Ellington. Although she did not have any Ellington records with her, she played some of the big band tunes she had on hand. Mr. Garcia listened passively. She left after about 30 minutes and said she would come to see him the next day.
>
> Upon her return, she played Mr. Garcia's favorite Ellington recording, "East St. Louis Toodle-oo." As it played, he began to move his hand in rhythm to the music. Ms. Reno handed him a drum mallet, which he grasped, and as she held a drum where he could reach it, Mr. Garcia began to play along with the music. At the conclusion of the selection she picked up a mallet, and as she began to play she asked him to join her. As they drummed together, she encouraged Mr. Garcia to play

in any manner that he would like, and modeled a few playing styles to guide him. When she played louder and stronger, so did he. Ms. Reno finally had to brace the drum against the side of the bed to withstand the force of his playing.

Ms. Reno allowed Mr. Garcia to continue to drum until he was exhausted. When he caught his breath, she said, "You sure seemed to beat out your frustrations!" He replied, "Well, I got a lot more, too!" "While you were drumming, you were frowning and your jaw looked really tight. How did you feel?" she asked. Mr. Garcia responded that he had felt miserable for a long time, but that the drumming made him feel a little better. Ms. Reno offered to come back the next day and Mr. Garcia said that he would like that.

Ms. Reno met daily with Mr. Garcia in a series of therapy sessions in which he beat the drum extremely loudly and forcefully. His drumming seemed to be a reflection of his emotions. As he continued to drum, Mr. Garcia began to express his thoughts and feelings. He talked about how he had tried to avoid losing his leg, but he could not bring his diabetes under control. He grieved over the loss of his leg and the terrible luck he felt he had. He spoke of how angry he was to have an illness over which he had no apparent control and for which there was no cure. He spoke of his fear of what might happen next in his life and of his concern that his friends might try to avoid him because they did not know what to say to him.

Mr. Garcia may have chosen not to speak of his feelings with Ms. Reno, but like other people who have had this experience, the rhythm provided the structure for expression. Rhythm creates a forum for sufficient emotional release, particularly for people who are not usually verbal about their feelings. Formal training is not necessary to participate in music in this way. The instruments that a person may use to participate include various styles and types of drums, claves, maracas, autoharps, and Omnichords. Professional-caliber instruments should be used because they produce the most pleasing sounds and people are more willing to commit to participate with these instruments than with poor-quality instruments. Instruments must be age appropriate and personally desirable or individuals will not attempt to play them.

Music therapy also provides opportunities for people who are geographically isolated or isolated by illness or fear to become acquainted, to pool their strengths in mutually satisfying ways, and to develop skills and abilities that facilitate successful musical experiences. The following vignette illustrates this concept:

> Marion and Belle were patients in a rehabilitation clinic following their strokes. They were withdrawn and had little social contact with staff or other patients. They were each approached by the facility's music therapist, who asked them if they would like to participate in music therapy. Both women were reluctant initially because they had no formal music training and could not use their left hands. The music therapist introduced them to one another and invited them to play an autoharp together. As Marion strummed the strings, Belle changed the chord buttons and the music therapist assisted. As the two women played the autoharp, the music therapist sang songs that were familiar to them. They joined in singing after they became adjusted to playing the instrument. The first session was so successful that Marion and Belle agreed to be scheduled for a joint music therapy session. Soon the women developed enough confidence to meet independent of the music therapist to practice playing and singing. They continued to attend music therapy to improve their musical skills and to learn new material.

Marion and Belle began performing for other patients, and the ladies' enthusiasm for the music encouraged them to participate in music as well. They also performed for their families and other visitors to the facility, which resulted in a larger support network for both of them.

PHYSICAL THERAPY FOR PEOPLE WITH
PARKINSON'S DISEASE

Parkinson's disease, or Parkinsonism (Parkinson, 1817), is a neurodegenerative disorder characterized by muscle tremor, rigidity, postural changes, and decreases in spontaneous movement that lead to bradykinesia (abnormal slowness of movement) and impairment of gait and postural stability (Greenberg, Aminoff, & Simon, 2002). Parkinson's disease is caused by a loss of dopamine-producing cells in the brain stem. The onset is insidious, progress is slow, and the full manifestation of symptoms occurs in later life (Greenberg et al., 2002). In addition to the physical symptoms, there is a strong indication that dementia eventually occurs in people in the advanced stages of the disease (Cedarbaum & McDowell, 1986).

People with Parkinson's disease have start hesitation (difficulty when beginning a stride) (Ambani & Van Woert, 1973). Once they begin a stride, they may take tiny steps and lean forward. This posture requires them to move increasingly faster. As they walk, their arms generally do not swing with the stride. If their arms do move, the excursion (range of motion) of the swing varies from one arm to the other (Greenberg et al., 2002). Posture is unstable as a result of decreased vestibular (of the ear) responses (Reichert, Doolittle, & McDowell, 1982; White, Saint-Cyr, & Sharpe, 1983) and decreased lower extremity reflexes (Traub, Rothwell, & Marsden, 1980). Consequently, balance is disturbed, weight distributions in the lower limbs are unequal, and gait is uneven or asymmetrical.

Parkinson's disease is incurable. The medication used to manage its symptoms is most effective on hypokinesia (abnormally decreased mobility) and bradykinesia. Postural instability is little (if at all) improved with medication. Over time, even the positive effects of medication diminish (Cedarbaum & McDowell, 1986). The need is great for nonpharmacological interventions that can ameliorate the symptoms associated with Parkinson's disease.

Using Music in Gait Training for People with Parkinson's Disease

Thaut and colleagues have investigated the effects of rhythmic auditory cueing by using music on the gait control of people with Parkinson's disease. They used a study model similar to the one they developed for gait training of people who had strokes. One experimental group and two control groups were studied. After 3 weeks, the experimental group, who used rhythmic auditory cueing for their at-home walking exercise program, had pronounced results. In comparing their pre- and posttests, which were completed without rhythmic auditory cueing, Thaut and colleagues found a 25% increase in walking efficiency. The subjects' step lengths, postural stability, rates of stepping, and electromyography of the lower limbs showed improvements in consistency and regularity. The first control group, which consisted of participants who exercised by walking without rhythmic auditory cueing, improved by only 7–8%. The second control group, comprised of persons who did not walk or receive rhythmic auditory cueing, showed no improvement at all at the conclusion of the 3-week study (McIntosh, Thaut, Rice, Miller, Rathbun, & Brault, 1995; Miller, Thaut, McIntosh, & Rice, 1996). Patients with Parkinson's disease who participated in a home-based program that used rhythmic auditory cueing significantly increased their gait velocity, stride length, and gait cadence (Thaut, McIntosh, Rice, Miller, Rathbun, & Brault, 1996).

Thaut (1994) suggests that rhythmic auditory cueing can be used successfully at home by people who want to maintain gait control. He recommends finding preferred music but cautions that the music must match the gait of the individual who wants to use it. Thaut explains that although a metronome is an effective rhythmic auditory cueing device, the best approach is to use music with clearly accented beats, which can serve as the external organizer for complex motor activities, such as walking.

The results of Thaut and colleagues' work are important to the restoration and maintenance of gait in people with Parkinson's disease. These clinical outcomes provide hope to people for whom management of the disease via medication is losing its effectiveness. Rhythmic auditory cueing enables people to achieve a rhythmic walking gait and stabilizes their posture, which is particularly important for people who lack the postural reflexes to correct imbalance using appropriate arm or leg movements. With rhythmic auditory cueing, these individuals are able to move forward using an appropriate stance, avoiding the propulsive gait that is used in an effort to remain upright. Rhythmic auditory cueing provides sufficient motor organization and control for these people to ambulate independently. However, cueing can become problematic if the source of the cue is disrupted. Thaut (1995) described a man who was elated with his restored independence and renewed ability to walk. He had developed such confidence during gait training and practice at home that one day he decided to walk alone to a local park with his portable audio player and headset. When he arrived at the park, which was a good distance from home, the batteries in the audio player died. Initially, he was panic-stricken as he realized how far he was from home and that his rhythmic gait depended on music. Once he calmed himself he decided that he would play the music mentally as he tried to walk home. After all, he thought, the music was familiar and he had used it successfully for some time. His ability to walk, he reasoned, was only a matter of allowing the music to play mentally to provide the rhythmic cues he needed. The man was able to walk home, moving to the music as it played at the appropriate tempo in his mind.

Oliver Sacks (*Forever Young: Music and Aging*, 1991) argued before the Senate Special Committee on Aging that the use of music in people with motor disorders and motor regulatory disorders was not a luxury but a necessity. This music, which he insisted must be preferred by them in order to be effective, promotes movement and is therefore essential to quality of life. He also described the responses of his patients with Parkinson's disease to music. One of his patients complained that the disease had taken music from her, that she had become "unmusicked." Her motor responses were no longer rhythmic and symmetrical, but when music was played in her environment, her rhythmic symmetry was restored. Another patient would sit transfixed all day until she played the piano, a skill she had acquired some years before. While she played, her movements were fluid, something not seen at any other time. Music transformed her when she played and when she was asked to recall it. In addition, an electroencephalogram taken of her brain activity showed normal activity as she imagined music, as opposed to her brain activity's almost coma-like slowness the remainder of the time.

Preliminary results of the study of the use of music with people with Parkinson's disease to organize motor responses, particularly responses associated with gait, show great promise. Using rhythmic auditory cues, people can maintain their independence and improve their quality of life. Any applications of music in ambulation must be selected carefully in order to match the motor skills and abilities of the person using it. Consultation with a physical therapist who is familiar with Thaut and colleagues' research concerning rhythmic auditory cueing is highly recommended.

AMBULATION REHABILITATION AFTER AMPUTATION

Of all amputations, approximately 75% are performed on people over age 65 years and are generally the result of ischemia (disruption in the arterial blood flow) (Studenski & Woods Duncan, 2004). The majority are lower limb amputations, and considerations for a prosthesis depend upon whether the individual is able to remove and attach the prosthesis independently, has good cardiopulmonary status along with good physical condition of the remaining limb, has a positive attitude, and was able to walk up until the time of the surgery (Steinberg, Garcia, Roettger, & Shelton, 1974).

When a prosthesis is recommended, rehabilitation is essential. It begins with the preparation of the stump and preprosthesis training, which includes full range of motion flexibility exercises for hip and knee joints three times a day (Stoner, 1971). Stump preparation and training are followed by prosthesis and ambulation training, which normally requires 2–3 weeks of residential care (Studenski & Woods Duncan, 2004).

Using Music in Ambulation Training with Lower Limb Prostheses

Although music therapists have not conducted specific research on the applications of music in ambulation training following amputation, information can be extrapolated from the studies of Thaut and colleagues concerning the use of rhythmic auditory cueing during gait training (explained in detail earlier in the chapter). The music must have accented, rhythmic beats, and the rhythmic beats must match the pace of the individual. Initially, the tempo used must be slow as the individual learns to incorporate his or her prosthesis into a walking gait. The pace can be increased as the tempo of the music is increased. Again, rhythm is the basis for organizing the stride symmetry from heel strike to heel strike. People with lower limb prosthesis may require an extended base of support, such as a quad (four-legged) cane, to provide stability. They must learn to incorporate an assistive device into their stride, which requires them to move the device in time with the stride on the side opposite the prosthetic limb. The assistive device is moved forward with the affected limb. To maximize a smooth gait, the entire movement must be completed in regular rhythm, and music can regulate the length and duration of each stride cycle.

CONCLUSION

Applications for therapeutic uses of music in health maintenance and rehabilitation have only begun to contribute to the quality of life of older adults. Continued efforts in clinical practice and research will build on the information on hand to further define possible applications of music therapy and their outcomes and benefits. To integrate music therapy into an exercise or physical rehabilitation program, consultation with a trained music therapist familiar with these applications is essential.

REFERENCES

Albert, M., Sparks, R., & Helm, N. (1973). Melodic intonation therapy for aphasics. *Archives of Neurology*, 29(2), 130–131.

Ambani, L. M., & Van Woert, M. H. (1973). Start hesitation—a side effect of long-term levodopa therapy. *New England Journal of Medicine*, 288(21), 1113.

American Heart Association. (2008). *Statistical fact sheet: Older Americans and cardiovascular disease–statistics*. Retrieved April 17, 2008, from http://www.americanheart.org/downloadable/heart/1199828277629FS08OLD8.REV.pdf

Andersson, A. G., Kamwendo, K., Seiger, A., & Appelros, P. (2006). How to identify potential fallers in a stroke unit: Validity indexes of 4 test methods. *Rehabilitation Medicine*, 38(1), 186–191.

Baker, F. A. (2000). Modifying the melodic intonation therapy program for adults with severe non-fluent aphasia. *Music Therapy Perspectives*, 18(2), 110–114.

Blumstein, S., & Cooper, W. (1974). Hemispheric processing of intonational contours. *Cortex*, 10, 146–158.

Bonakdarpour, B., Eftekharzadeh, A., & Ashayeri, H. (2000). Preliminary report on the effects of melodic intonation therapy in the rehabilitation of Persian aphasic patients. *Iranian Journal of Medical Sciences*, 25, 156–160.

Broussard, D. L., & Altschuler, S. M. (2000). Central integration of swallow and airway-protective relexes. *American Journal of Medicine*, 108(4A), 62S–67S.

Cedarbaum, J. M., & McDowell, G. H. (1986). Sixteen-year follow up of 100 patients begun on levodopa in 1968: Emerging problems. *Advances in Neurology*, 45, 469–472.

Chaudhuri, G., Hildner, C., Brady, S., Hutchins, B., Aliga, N., & Abadilla, E. (2002). Cardiovascular effects of the supraglottic and super-supraglottic swallowing maneuvers in stroke patients with dysphagia. *Dysphagia*, 17(1), 19–23.

Clair, A. A., & O'Konski, M. (2006). The effect of rhythmic auditory stimulation (RAS) on gait characteristics of cadence, velocity, and stride length in persons with late stage dementia. *Journal of Music Therapy*, 43(2), 154–163.

Cohen, N. S. (1992). The effect of singing instruction on the speech production of neurologically impaired persons. *Journal of Music Therapy*, 29(2), 82–107.

Cohen, N. S., & Masse, R. (1993). The application of singing and rhythmic instruction as a therapeutic intervention for persons with neurogenic communication disorders. *Journal of Music Therapy*, 30(2), 81–99.

Confrancesco, E. (1985). The effect of music therapy on hand grasp strength and functional task performance in stroke patients. *Journal of Music Therapy*, 22(3), 129–145.

Cooper, J. J., & Glassow, R. B. (1982). *Kinesiology*. St. Louis, MO: C. V. Mosby.

Digenio, A. G., Sim, J. G., Krige, K., Stewart, A., Morris, R., Dowdeswell, R. J., & Padaychee, G. N. (1991). The Johannesburg cardiac rehabilitation programme. *South African Medical Journal*, 79(4), 183–187.

Dishman, R. K. (1982). Compliance/adherence in health-related exercise. *Health Psychology*, 1(3), 237–267.

Dorland's illustrated medical dictionary (29th ed.). (2000). Philadelphia: W. B. Saunders.

Duncan, W., Weiner, D., Chandler, J., & Studenski, S. (1990).

Functional reach: A new clinical measure of balance. *Journal of Gerontology: Medical Sciences*, 45(6), M192–M197.

Edelberg, H. K. (2004). Assessment of the geriatric patient. In D. C. Dale & D. D. Federman (Eds.), *ACP medicine* (Section 75, pp. 943–948). New York: WebMD Professional Publishing.

Forever young: Music and aging: Hearings before the Senate Special Committee on Aging, 102d Cong. 1st Sess. 13 (1991). (Testimony of Oliver Sacks).

Goldie, P. A., Evans, O. M., & Bach, T. M. (1992). Steadiness in one-legged stance: Development of a reliable force-platform testing procedure. *Archives of Physical Medicine & Rehabilitation*, 73(4), 348–354.

Greenberg, D., Aminoff, M. J., & Simon, R. P. (2002). *Clinical neurology* (5th ed.). Columbus: McGraw-Hill.

Hanser, S. B., & Mandel, S. E. (2005). The effects of music therapy in cardiac healthcare. *Cardiology in Review*, 13(1), 18–23.

Hayden, R., Clair, A. A., Johnson, G., & Otto, D. (2007). *The effects of rhythmic auditory stimulation (RAS) on clinical outcomes in a wait-listed control study of patients with recent stroke*. Unpublished manuscript, The University of Kansas, Lawrence.

Holohan-Bell, J. K., & Brummel-Smith, K. (1999). Impaired mobility and deconditioning. In J. T. Stone, J. F. Wyman, & S. A. Salisbury (Eds.), *Clinical gerontologial nursing: A guide to advanced practice* (2nd ed.) (pp. 267–288). Philadelphia: W. B. Saunders.

Huff, J. (1972). Auditory and visual perception of rhythm by performers skilled in selected motor activities. *Research Quarterly*, 43(2), 197–207.

Jeong, S., & Kim, M. T. (2007). Effect of a theory-driven music and music program for stroke survivors in a community setting. *Applied Nursing Research*, 20(3), 125–131.

Kim, S. (2006). *The effect of music therapy to enhance swallowing training for stroke patients with dysphagia.* Unpublished manuscript, University of Kansas at Lawrence.

Kisner, C., & Colby, L. A. (2007). *Therapeutic exercise: Foundations and techniques* (5th ed.). Philadelphia: F. A. Davis.

Krauss, T., & Galloway, H. (1982). Melodic intonation therapy with language delayed, apraxic children. *Journal of Music Therapy*, 19(2), 102–113.

Laughlin, S. A., Naeser, M. A., & Gordon, W. P. (1979). Effects of three syllable durations using the melodic intonation therapy technique. *Journal of Speech and Hearing Research*, 22(2), 311–320.

Lhamon, W. T., & Goldstone, S. (1974). Studies of auditory-visual differences in human time judgment. II: More transmitted information with sounds than lights. *Perceptual and Motor Skills*, 39(1), 295–307.

Logemann, J. A. (1995). Dysphagia: Evaluation and treatment. *Folia Phoniatrica Logopedia*, 47(3), 140–164.

Luft, A. R., McCombe-Waller, S., Whitall, J., Forrester, L. W., Macko, R., Sorkin, J. D., Schulz, J. B, Goldberg, A. P., & Hanley, D. F. (2004). Repetitive bilateral arm training and motor cortex activation in chronic stroke: A randomized controlled trial. *Journal of the American Medical Association*, 292(15), 1853–1861.

MacNay, S. K. (1995). The influence of preferred music on the perceived exertion, mood, and time estimation scores of patients participating in a cardiac rehabilitation exercise program. *Music Therapy Perspectives*, 13(2), 91–96.

Mandel, S. E. (1996). Music for wellness: Music therapy for stress management in a rehabilitation program. *Music Therapy Perspectives*, 14(1), 38–43.

McIntosh, G., Thaut, M., Rice, R., Miller, R., Rathbun, J., & Brault, J. (1995). Rhythmic facilitation in gait training of Parkinson's disease. *Annals of Neurology*, 38, 331.

Mendelsohn, M. S., & Martin, R. E. (1993). Airway protection during breath-holding. *Annals of Otology, Rhinology, & Laryngology*, 102(12), 941–944.

Metzger, L. K. (2004). Assessment of use of music by patients participating in cardiac rehabilitation. *Journal of Music Therapy*, 41(1), 55–69.

Miller, R., Thaut, M., McIntosh, C., & Rice, R. (1996). Components of EMG symmetry and variability in Parkinsonian and healthy elderly gait. *Electroencephalography and Clinical Neurophysiology*, 101(1), 1–7.

Murrock, C. J. (2002). The effects of music on the rate of perceived exertion and general mood among coronary artery bypass graft patients enrolled in cardiac rehabilitation phase II. *Rehabilitation Nursing*, 27(6), 227–231.

Pal'tsev, U. I., & El'ner, A. M. (1967). Change in the functional state of the segmental apparatus of the spinal cord under the influence of sound stimuli and its role in voluntary movement. *Biophysics*, 12, 1219–1226.

Parkinson, J. (1817). *An essay on the shaking palsy*. London: Sherwood, Neely & Jones.

Perry, L. (2001). Screening swallowing function of patients with acute stroke. Part one: Identification, implementation and initial evaluation of a screening tool for use by nurses. *Journal of Clinical Nursing*, 10(4), 463–473.

Prassas, S. G., Thaut, M. H., McIntosh, G. C., & Rice, R. R. (1997). Effect of auditory rhythm cueing on gait kinematic parameters in stroke patients. *Gait and Posture*, 6(3), 218–223.

Reichert, W. H., Doolittle, J., & McDowell, F. H. (1982). Vestibular dysfunction in Parkinson's disease. *Neurology*, 32(4), 1133–1138.

Reuben, D., Laliberte, L., Hiris, J., & Mor, V. (1990). A hierarchical exercise scale to measure function at the advanced activities of daily living (AADL) level. *Journal of the American Geriatric Society*, 38(8), 855–861.

Rochester, L., Hetherington, V., Jones, D., Nieuwboer, A., Willems, A., Kwakkel, G., & Van Wegen, E. (2005). The effect of external rhythmic cues (auditory and visual) on walking during a functional task in homes of people with Parkinson's disease. *Archives of Physical Medicine and Rehabilitation*, 86(5), 999–1006.

Rossignol, S., & Melville Jones, C. (1976). Audio-spinal influence in man studied by the H-reflex and its possible role on rhythmic movement synchronized to sound. *Electroencephalography and Clinical Neurophysiology*, 41(1), 83–92.

Rozanski, A., & Blumenthal, J. (2006). Cardiac rehabilitation, exercise training, and psychosocial risk factors: Reply. *Journal of the American College of Cardiology*, 47(1), 212–213.

Rubenstein, T. C., Giladi, N., & Hausdorff, J. M. (2002). The power of cueing to circumvent dopamine deficits: A review of physical therapy treatment of gait disturbances in Parkinson's disease. *Movement Disorders*, 17(6), 1148–1160.

Seiger, J. E., & Hirschfeld, H. (2004). One-leg stance in healthy young and elderly adults: A measure of postural steadiness? *Clinical Biomechanics*, 19, 688–694.

Sparks, R. W., Helm, N., & Albert, M. (1974). Aphasia rehabilitation resulting from melodic intonation therapy, *Cortex*, 10(4), 313–316.

Sparks, R. W., & Holland, A. L. (1976). Method: Melodic intonation therapy for aphasia. *Journal of Speech and Hearing Disorders*, 41(3), 287–297.

Staum, M. (1983). Music and rhythmic stimuli in the rehabilitation of gait disorders. *Journal of Music Therapy*, 29(2), 69–87.

Steinberg, F., Garcia, W., Roettger, R., & Shelton, D. (1974). Rehabilitation of the geriatric amputee. *Journal of the American Geriatrics Society*, 22(2), 62–66.

Stoner, E. K. (1971). Management of the lower extremity amputee. In F. J. Kottke, G. K. Stillwell, & J. F. Lehmann (Eds.), *Handbook of physical medicine and rehabilitation* (3rd ed.) (p. 921). Philadelphia: W. B. Saunders.

Studenski, S., & Woods Duncan, P. (2004). Rehabilitation of geriatric patients. In D. C. Dale & D. D. Federman (Eds.), *ACP medicine* (Section 77, pp. 970–980). New York: WebMD Professional Publishing.

Thaut, M. (1988). Rhythmic intervention techniques in music therapy with gross motor dysfunctions. *Arts in Psychotherapy*, 15(2), 127–137.

Thaut, M. (1994). *Rhythmic sensorimotor music therapy for gait training with Parkinson's disease patients* [Video]. (Available from the Office of Instructional Service, Colorado State University, Fort Collins, CO 80523)

Thaut, M. (1995, March). *Rhythmic auditory cueing in Parkinson's disease patients*. Paper presented at the Midwestern regional annual conference of the National Association for Music Therapy, Fort Collins, CO.

Thaut, M. (1999). *Training manual for neurologic music therapy*. Fort Collins, CO: Center for Biomedical Research in Music, Colorado State University.

Thaut, M., & McIntosh, G. (1992). Effect of auditory rhythm on temporal stride parameters and EMG patterns in normal and hemiparetic gait [Abstract]. *Neurology*, 42(Suppl. 3), 208.

Thaut, M., McIntosh, G., Prassas, S., & Rice, R. (1992a). Effect of auditory rhythmic pacing on normal gait and gait in stroke, cerebellar disorder, and transverse myelitis. In M. Woollacott & E. Horak (Eds.), *Posture and gait: Control mechanisms* (pp. 437–440). Eugene, OR: University of Oregon Books.

Thaut, M., McIntosh, G., Prassas, S., & Rice, R. (1992b). Effect of rhythmic auditory cuing on temporal stride parameters and EMG patterns in normal gait. *Journal of Neurological Rehabilitation*, 6, 185–190.

Thaut, M., McIntosh, G., Prassas, S., & Rice, R. (1993). The effect of auditory rhythmic cuing on stride and EMG patterns in hemiparetic gait of stroke patients. *Journal of Neurologic Rehabilitation*, 7(1), 9–16.

Thaut, M. H., McIntosh, G. C., & Rice, R. R. (1997). Rhythmic facilitation of gait training in hemiparetic stroke rehabilitation. *Journal of Neurological Science*, 151, 207–212.

Thaut, M., McIntosh, G., Rice, R., Miller, R., Rathbun, J., & Brault, J. (1996). Rhythmic auditory stimulation in gait training for Parkinson's disease patients. *Movement Disorders*, 11(2), 193–200.

Thomas, J. R., & Moon, D. H. (1976). Measuring motor rhythmic ability in children. *Research Quarterly*, 47(1), 20–32.

Traub, M. M., Rothwell, J. C., & Marsden, C. D. (1980). Anticipatory postural reflexes in Parkinson's disease and other akinetic-rigid syndromes and in cerebellar ataxia. *Brain*, 103(2), 393.

Tsunoda, K., Aikawa, J., Murakami, R., Sakai, Y., & Kikkawa, Y. (2003). Bent (head-down) posture and aberrant internal carotid artery in the mouth: A new risk factor for stroke? *Annals of Internal Medicine*, 139(1), W-56.

Tsunoda, K., Ishimoto, S., Aikawa, J., Shinogrami, M., Murakami, R., Saigusa, H., Kondou, K., & Bitou, S. (2005). Bent (head-down) posture and aberrant common carotid arteries of the neck: Another new risk factor for stroke? *Laryngoscope*, 115(11), 2074–2075.

White, O. B., Saint-Cyr, R. D., & Sharpe, J. A. (1983). Ocular motor deficits in Parkinson's disease. I: The horizontal vestibulo-ocular reflex and its regulation. *Brain*, 106(3), 555.

Wilson, S. J., Parsons, K., & Reutens, D. C. (2006). Preserved singing in aphasia: A case study of the efficacy of melodic intonation therapy. *Music Perception*, 2(1), 23–26.

Chapter 9

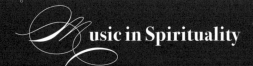

Music in Spirituality

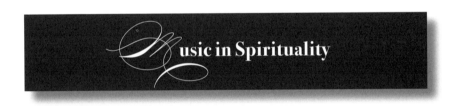

Music has always been used in religious practices. Merriam (1964) explained that one of the functions of music is to validate social institutions and religious rituals. Thus, music is used to retell myths and legends in song and to express religious precepts. Music may also be incorporated into religious practices to enhance prayer, express feelings, focus attention, mask distractions, and establish a context for ritual. Above all, music draws people together for a common purpose (Gaston, 1968). Having accomplished this, music provides a framework for group participation through rhythm and familiarity.

It is the music and the context for religious practices that constitute the external structures and expectations for religious behaviors. Although these religious practices may be among the ways in which spirituality is externally expressed by some people, spirituality and religion are not synonymous. *Spirituality* is an internal state of being that goes beyond external forms of expression and involves experience with a deity, god, or higher power. However, it is conceptualized by an individual. *Religion* is the traditional forms and practices associated with spirituality that provide access to the deity, god, or higher power (herein referred to as "God").

Spirituality means different things to different people, and it can have different meanings for people at various times in their lives. Some older people become interested in confirming or developing their spirituality. Often, they wish to contemplate the meaning of their life and to find peace and contentment in their daily existence. They wish to reach beyond the physical conditions of this world to achieve a sense of wholeness, well-being, and belonging. They seek solace in God when supernatural assistance is needed in order to endure the unknown, to live and work through life's losses, and to experience renewed hope for the future. However, it is erroneous to assume that all older people want to explore spiritual matters. It also should never be assumed that spiritual pursuits must follow a particular path. The interest, need, or desire for spirituality must come from within the individual and must be expressed in ways that are appropriate to, or compatible with, the individual's cultural background, belief system, and personal experience.

THE NEED FOR SPIRITUALITY

The need for spirituality must be individually defined. It can range from the need for deeper calm, peace, and serenity to a frantic need for a way to manage pain, fear, or anxiety. The spiritual journey to meet these needs usually begins with the realization that the fulfillment of physical desires does not necessarily lead to happiness and contentment. For some, the journey is a natural continuation of a life already involved in the development of their faith (Fowler, 1995). Others begin their spiritual journey resulting from their own catastrophic illness or disability in an attempt to relieve their fear of that over which they have little or no control. For others, the need for spirituality comes from the need to heal from experiencing loss and other emotional afflictions.

Loss has a tremendous impact on human life and takes many forms. Initially, loss is recognized as physical changes (e.g., changes in endurance, flexibility, strength, agility) that begin in midlife. These changes are all part of normal aging and may worsen every year. Losses in physical function may be accompanied by the emotional losses associated with lifestyle changes resulting from sickness, disability, divorce, or death. As people age, these losses happen more frequently and may become progressively difficult to endure. The news of yet another death or divorce is stressful, and feelings of abandonment often follow. People who feel abandoned by the death or divorce of friends or loved ones often reflect on their own vulnerability. Such reflection can raise fears of the future, including possible loneliness, isolation, lingering illness, an absence of caregivers, pain and suffering, and death. Often, individuals seek spiritual comfort to assuage these fears.

Although the fear of death is strong in some people, it may be superseded by the fear of physical pain and disability so severe that circumstances necessitate supervised health care and a subsequent loss of independence. Supervised health care can range from home health care to placement in a residential care facility. Residential placement is necessary when it is no longer safe for a physically frail, chronically ill, or cognitively impaired individual to live at home. The losses associated with the move that are experienced by the new resident range from a sense of failure to maintain physical or cognitive integrity to a loss of social involvement and subsequent isolation.

Some residents question why they are still living when many of their friends and family members are gone. They may have few people (in some cases, no one) with whom to share a sense of belonging, and they may be too frail or grief-stricken to reach out to others to establish new relationships. For many older individuals, spiritual activities can provide a sense of belonging to and acceptance by other people and their God.

Caregivers (e.g., spouse, adult children, friend, other family member) may also experience loss associated with residential care placement. Their losses come from changing roles and the prolonged absence of people who have been a central part of their lives. Caregivers become visitors in residential care facilities. Although they may integrate themselves into facility care regimens on some level, the type of involvement changes and their roles are assumed by the nursing staff. Often, caregivers experience guilt for having turned over the total care of loved ones to others. This guilt and other changes associated with residential care placement can erode the relationship between caregivers and care recipients. To prevent this erosion, some caregivers struggle to ingratiate themselves with their loved ones via frequent visits and frequent interactions with nursing staff and administrators. Other caregivers do not face the changes and withdraw from their loved ones, particularly if those loved ones have deteriorated severely from a progressive dementia. Caregivers may feel they have failed in some or many ways. They may feel helpless, unable to cope, and empty because of the absence of the loved one. To resolve these feelings, caregivers may seek spiritual comfort.

Feelings of loss are also associated with people's unrealized dreams and the disappointment that accompanies them. When it becomes apparent (as a result of a lack of physical strength, time, energy, money, or other resources) that the dreams are inaccessible and will never become reality, the dreams must end. The death of a dream is a valid source of grief. It represents the end of hope for a future long planned and imagined. People need to grieve and heal emotionally and spiritually from the losses associated with unrealized dreams. These needs are no less real than the need to recover from other losses, and one's spirituality may provide comfort.

Some individuals accept aging with tranquility. They seem

fully conscious of the changes that aging brings. These older people have strong feelings of loss and grief, yet they adjust more readily to change than people who do not easily accept aging. They do not seem to fear the unknown and respond to it by participating fully in making adaptations.

For example, moving to a residential care facility may provide relief from the stresses and worries associated with providing self-care or care to others. Some people may experience stress from the actual move, but the knowledge that they are moving to a facility where they will receive professional care gives them peace of mind that may override the stress.

Many older people speak of appreciating moments, hours, or days in which they feel well and at peace, and say they will "do what they have to do" when their well-being is altered by events beyond their control. Their need for a spiritual journey comes from the desire to maintain their acceptance, peace, and contentment as circumstances in and around them change. The following vignette illustrates the adaptive capabilities of one woman in the face of loss:

> One woman described her recent widowhood as a matter of course, but also as a terrible loss: "I always thought I'd be by myself one day. All my friends are widowed and my husband had been very sick for some time. I am so thankful that he died quickly and that it was not too difficult for either him or me. I know that all things work together for good, and his death was like that, too. I think about all the happy times we had, and I miss him terribly. He used to do so many thoughtful things for me. I really didn't realize how much, until he was gone. I fully expected to be alone eventually, and I have my moments when I cry, but I'm all right."

THE SPIRITUAL JOURNEY

The goal of spiritual growth is oneness with God (Peck, 2003). People who have achieved this goal seem well able to let go, to surrender to God, and to experience God's power. They live each day confident that they are united with the divine. People who have not achieved the goal attempt to control everything. They have a high level of anxiety and rely on external behaviors, or rituals, in an effort to manage it. These individuals strive to employ the correct ritual using the appropriate numbers of repetitions in the proper combination and sequence with other rituals. They have little faith that their needs and desires will be met, and they doubt their worth as individuals. When they do not receive what they desire, they blame the structure of the ritual or their inability to use the correct ritual in the correct way. They accept total responsibility for failure and assume that their lack of true worth is the reason for their lack of fulfillment.

Individuals may become anxious, agitated, compulsive, and even obsessive in their efforts to develop their spiritual lives when they conceptualize God as a punitive being, particularly as a parent figure. These responses are sometimes traced to a history of threats, physical abuse, neglect, or even incest. As a result, these individuals have developed defensive and protective behaviors that incorporate control of self and others. Within this context, it is difficult for them to consider letting go of these behaviors, even when these behaviors have led to isolation and loneliness. It is also difficult for them to release this control in order to experience God.

People who are confident in their faith may involve themselves in religious rituals that provide them with a connection to traditional values and other people who have practiced these rituals. They find solace in those values and in the familiarity provided by the rituals, while using the rituals to achieve deeper experiences with God. Therefore, these rituals are not performed merely as social or cultural protocol, but as an opportunity for deep spiritual fulfillment.

Clearly, spirituality does not happen spontaneously. It requires effort, constant attention, and the performance of certain activities that keep spiritual principles and understandings alive (Moore, 1992). Spirituality is, therefore, an ongoing process that begins with a desire to become one with God and evolves into a progressively more intimate experience with God. Often, the desire is actualized initially by overt, active behaviors, such as praying, gestures (e.g., kneeling, hands folded in prayer), singing, playing an instrument, dancing, meeting in groups, creating works of visual and dramatic arts, studying sacred writings, and seeking testimony or spiritual direction from others with more experience and maturity in spiritual matters, that focus attention and heighten awareness.

As individuals decide to change their locus of control and as they mature in their spiritual lives, they may engage in less overt expressive behaviors. They may become contemplative, involving themselves frequently in quiet meditation with God (*The Cloud of Unknowing*, 1979). Contemplation contributes to spiritual development because it is quiet time away from the cares, concerns, and activities of the world. The place for contemplation may be any place where quiet solitude is possible, such as a space in one's home or in one's room at a residential care facility, a synagogue, a church, a library, an art gallery, or a garden.

Some people describe their times of greatest closeness with God when sitting alone, their minds emptied of all concerns. They may have little awareness of their surroundings, but they feel a deep sense of contentment and well-being. It is a feeling that can come only from silent contemplation.

People who derive personal benefit from quiet time alone may also participate in religious rituals that afford opportunities to meet with others who share traditional beliefs and practices. They draw support from their communities as they attempt to grow spiritually. They may also seek direction from a spiritual leader. They feel comfortable and confident that they are moving toward life-enhancing experiences with God.

Some people draw strength from being alone with God, whereas other people may experience God more intimately in the presence of others. Other experiences alone, coupled with some experiences in the company of others, bring them closer to God.

USING MUSIC TO ENHANCE SPIRITUALITY

Music can enhance spirituality when used in prayer and religious ritual.

Using Music in Prayer

The word *prayer* comes from the Latin *precari*, which means to entreat or implore and to address God with adoration, confession, supplication, or thanksgiving. Prayer can be a petition for oneself or an intercession for another. In any form, prayer is a connection to God and provides affirmation of immortality, awareness of an eternal presence, and assurance that one is not alone (Dossey, 1997). Prayer may be directed, undirected, silent, or audible, and music may be used to facilitate it. Songs and instrumental music, whether composed or improvised, may be used to draw attention from this world to the divine power of God.

To use music to focus prayer, it is important to consider the frames of mind, activity levels, and emotional states of those wishing to pray. Individuals who are anxious or agitated may find it difficult to surrender themselves to prayer, although they may wish to do so. Music that matches their emotional state and a text that relates to the purpose of the prayer may initiate the process. The music may begin with quick tempos and be progressively altered to include less rapid tempos, longer phrases, and more solemn texts as individuals calm and focus their attention. Although some people require music that is progressively sedative to settle into prayer, others in similar emotional states may calm quickly upon hearing or performing music they associate with prayer. Certain hymns or chants may cue them to begin praying and to enter a state of mind in which the worries and concerns of the world are blotted out.

Some forms of prayer are quiet and solemn, whereas others are filled with sound and activity. Spoken prayers with shouts and gestures (e.g., waving, gyrating movements, clapping, stomping) may be desirable. Music reflects the form of prayer with rapid tempos, syncopated rhythms, and lyrics. This type of prayer usually begins quietly and becomes progressively louder and more animated. The music matches the level of activity, beginning with a sedative quality with regular rhythms, smooth melodic contours, and lyrics that set the tone for what is to come. As prayer grows louder and more active, so does the music. Rhythms become accented and syncopated, and melodies may be improvised or contain percussive characteristics. Responses to the music by participants are physically active and may seem out of control, but the music manages behavior by providing structure. As the tempo, syncopation, and volume of the music increase, the physical activity, emotional expression, and vocal responses of the participants also increase. When it is time to return to calm and quiet, the music gradually settles back to regular rhythms and smooth melodic contours.

Music itself may also be a form of prayer. The music may include traditional or newly composed songs with texts based in sacred writings or chants without any discernible words. The music may also be instrumental, either composed expressly for use in prayer or completely improvised. Whether the music is traditional, chosen specifically by individuals, or newly composed, it demonstrates a personal commitment to prayer. This type of music selection and performance reaches out to God and forms the basis of an experience with God.

Using Music in Religious Ritual

Rituals give form to human life (Campbell & Fairchild, 1993) and religious rituals provide a form within which prayer and experience with God may take place. Rituals may be conducted by individuals while alone, or they may be implemented within a community of people. They may include certain conventions with extensive histories, or they may consist of innovative practices designed to reawaken interest in worship.

Rituals have several components that generally occur in a particular order. The components of a ritual may be altered to increase or decrease its length, but most often all components are included each time the ritual is performed. Among these components are gathering, focusing on divine power, listening to religious teachings, affirming beliefs, petitioning, offering, receiving communion, and thanksgiving and dismissal.

The components of a ritual may be accompanied by music. The musical selections and the ways in which they are performed may be traditional or they may be new songs or instrumental music. Whatever the source of the music, it is intended to heighten the ritual experience. Most importantly, music draws people together and helps to create an integrated community. It enhances their awareness of being with others who share their most important values. Music facilitates a sense of belonging, which is essential to personal well-being.

Gathering

The first component of a ritual is the gathering. Gathering may mean physically bringing together a group of individuals or bringing an individual's attention to a point of focus. In addition, an individual may feel a closeness to other people who have participated in the ritual in the past or to those who practice the ritual elsewhere (e.g., another community, a different house of worship). The purpose of the gathering may be a celebration of the beginning or the end of life, a celebration of hopefulness, a demonstration of mutual concern and support, or healing of pain and suffering. Song lyrics reflect these purposes as they focus the attention of the participants. The tonality, rhythm, and tempo of the music reflect feelings: faster tempos with accented beats and major tonalities generally indicate feelings of joy and celebration. Slower tempos with few or no accented beats and minor tonalities generally indicate more somber occasions.

Focusing on Divine Power

After people gather, music focuses their attention on the power of God and helps them to acknowledge their frailty and to ask God for mercy, understanding, and forgiveness. Music expresses what cannot be expressed in words and promotes involvement through active participation or emotional responses. Again, song lyrics and the general presentation of musical elements (e.g., melody, rhythm, timbre, and tonality) heighten the experience of rituals and the outward expressions of feelings associated with them. Therefore, it is essential that music selections be appropriate to the purpose of the ritual.

Listening to Religious Teachings

Religious teachings are derived from traditional religious writings and impart the values and purpose of a spiritual life. These writings are used to provide direction for behavior and comfort. The teachings may be preceded by prayers, songs, or chants that raise an individual's consciousness and open his or her heart to the power of God and the importance of the teachings. Often, the teachings are followed by their interpretation and contemporary application as delivered by a religious leader. Some moments of silent reflection may follow, which allow individuals to assimilate the message into their own lives.

Affirming Beliefs

Rituals include an acknowledgment of the power of God. This acknowledgment takes the form of recited principles of belief, which are offered with respect, praise, and thanksgiving. Songs and prayers focus participants' attention on God's power and the participants' faith that this power exists and works for the common good.

Petitioning

Once centered on God's power and the strength of that power, participants offer petitions for people in need. These petitions are offered either publicly or silently by the congregation, and they are made with faith that the needs can be met. Petitions may include pleas to heal the sick, to help people who serve others (e.g., missionaries), to protect individuals from harm (e.g., evil influences, damaging weather), and to provide for daily needs. The prayers and the songs that accompany the petitions reflect the faith and confidence that the requests will be filled.

Offering

Rituals may include an offering, such as goods, services, money, materials, or self, to God. The offering may be accompanied by instrumental music or song. Music itself may constitute an offering. The offering is made with humility in recognition of the power of God and is accompanied by prayers and songs that affirm the benevolence of God.

Receiving Communion

The ritual may include a communion ceremony, described by Moore (1992) as a metaphor for union with God, in which taking food and drink into the body is a way of absorbing God into oneself. Religions or individuals who do not take part in communion may chant, sing, or pray silently. These methods help individuals to confess their human frailties, open themselves to God, acclaim the goodness and the power of God, and surrender to God's power.

Thanksgiving and Dismissal

Before the conclusion of the ritual, there may be a time of quiet contemplation and prayer. This quiet time is used to focus consciousness on the purpose and the importance of the ritual and to offer thanksgiving to God. It is a time to speak from the heart and to renew individual commitments to God. It is also a time to become peaceful before leaving the ritual. When this time of contemplation concludes, music provides closure to the ritual. This music guides activity and behaviors at closure and after closure, and provides a sense of security, predictability, and familiarity. Participants are sent away from the ritual having had a common experience, which engenders a sense of belonging. This feeling of inclusion may be accompanied by a renewed sense of vigor and hope. The melody and words of the final song and the music played or sung as people leave the gathering reflect these feelings and are associated with them throughout the hours and days that follow.

Importance of Using Music in Ritual

Music is integrated into all components of a ritual and directly reflects all the feelings associated with the occasion (e.g., solemnity, reverence, joy, sadness). Music also heightens the experience of these feelings. It seems that without music, rituals lose much of their potency—anniversaries and weddings seem less festive and funerals seem too morbid and empty. Music not only heightens the experiences of the feelings within the ritual but also evokes the feelings when the music is heard or performed outside the ritual. These feelings are as real as those experienced during the religious ritual. It is therefore possible for people to use this music outside the ritual to evoke feelings associated with the ritual and then to worship (e.g., through prayer). The music can enhance a state of mind or a feeling that leads to greater spiritual awareness both inside and outside the context of ritual.

USING MUSIC IN MEDITATION

To meditate is to engage in contemplation or reflection. This may be accomplished by focusing on a particular image or concept or by emptying the mind of thoughts and images (Naranjo, 1979). Whatever the approach, the thoughts and pressures of the day are set aside while one focuses on spirituality. This focus allows one to relinquish control and to achieve tranquility. However, the process of relinquishing control can be frightening in initial meditation experiences, and using music may be desirable to provide a predictable, external structure. Music can be used to enhance meditation by focusing individuals' attention and awareness and by blocking intrusive and distracting thoughts, preoccupations, and concerns. With more experience, it may be unnecessary or even undesirable to use music after inducing meditation.

Although music can contribute to meditation, music can also detract from it, especially music that is associated with unrelated events, memories, or activities. When selecting music as a meditation facilitator, one must consider the extramusical associations it may have and actually test the music to determine whether it has effects that contribute to or detract from its purpose. Associations that contribute to the purpose may include memories of occasions when a particular song evoked comfort. People may also associate music with images, such as an image of a loving God who encircles them with gentle, strong, and protective arms during meditation. Other people using the same music may see images of loneliness and abandonment (e.g., because the music was featured at a parent's funeral). Having such negative associations, the music inhibits the meditation process and is therefore contraindicated for these individuals.

Because associations with music are based on individual experiences and can either distract from or contribute to meditation, each person who wishes to use music in meditation must select the most appropriate music for him or her. Making the selection is best accomplished by listening to entire pieces of music to determine personal reactions to them. Music that evokes any discomfort or harmful reactions must not be used. Using music in meditation groups is not as effective because it is impossible to select music that will enhance the meditative experience of all participants. Even if there is agreement among members of the group that a certain type of music is satisfactory, it will not be as productive for some people as it is for others.

Inducing Meditation

Individuals who wish to meditate must begin by placing themselves in a quiet state in which they can disassociate themselves from the concerns and events of the world and focus on spiritual matters for a period of time. The amount of time can vary, depending on the desires and the physical, emotional, social, and psychological constraints of the individual. Initially, this quiet state may be difficult to achieve, especially when an individual is caught up in the pressures and events of the day or is feeling depressed, hurt, anxious, remorseful, or preoccupied. In order for individuals to meditate, they must focus their attention. One way to achieve this state is through music.

Music helps individuals to place themselves in a meditative state by imposing a rhythmic framework that provides order and structure. Provided this framework matches the mood and activity level of the participants, they will respond to it by organizing their responses to fit within the predictable, secure context. These responses can be altered as the music is altered, provided the changes are not extreme and do not occur too rapidly. Matching the music to suit individuals' moods and activity levels is best accomplished by asking them how they feel and by observing their behaviors carefully. If an individual typically has active thoughts that intrude on efforts to sit or lie quietly or to concentrate on a specific idea, music having quick tempos, definitely accented beats, syncopated rhythms, and melodies with major tonalities should be selected. Gradually, the music selections are sequenced from those having rapid tempos with accented beats to slower tempos that have no accented beats or syncopations. This progression is designed to encourage individuals to focus their attention from the intrusions of the day to an opportunity for peace. If an individual typically is lethargic and apathetic, music having slow tempos, regular beats that are generally unaccented, and melodies with minor tonalities must be used. The music selections for this individual are gradually sequenced from those having minor tonality to selections having major tonality. Throughout the transition in tonality, the music maintains regular, unaccented rhythms and slow tempos to promote quiet and calm and to focus the individual on the induction process.

Induction may be further enhanced by using a mantra, which is a word or phrase selected by an individual. The mantra is chanted repeatedly, either mentally or aloud (Ornstein, 1979). Chanting a mantra slows breathing and increases the breath volume while directing a person's attention to a desirable idea or state of mind. Instead of, or in addition to a mantra, an individual may focus attention on a mandala, which can be defined as a visual image of a circle, or some other form (Ornstein, 1979). The mandala serves to eliminate thoughts that detract from the meditation experience. The images within the mandala may be anything the individual desires, such as the face of God.

As the music plays, individuals' breathing patterns adjust to the rhythm of the music. Eventually, breathing becomes slow and deep. If singing or chanting is not desirable, individuals may breathe deeply in time to the music. This focus on breathing helps to direct attention away from individuals' concerns and worries, and the increased oxygenation in conjunction with biochemical changes that occur in the body in response to music produce beneficial effects in mood (Thaut, 2005).

Whatever device is used to induce meditation—mantras, mandalas, or music alone, caution must be exercised because some people believe that these approaches are evil. These individuals believe that they provoke evil influences in the world, and that these approaches must never be a part of spiritual practice. Therefore, it is important to determine an individual's religious practices before any meditative approach is attempted.

The Meditative State

Meditation helps people to transcend ordinary life experiences in order to reach a state of unconditional acceptance and well-being that can be euphoric. This process of transcendence may or may not incorporate music, but when music is used, it generally has a slow tempo with regular, unaccented, unsyncopated beats. Often without lyrics, the melodies used in this phase of the meditation process are smooth and contain little melodic variation. Because the music structures the experience, the individual can relax into progressively deeper levels of meditation. People can do this with confidence that the music will continue through time in a predictable way and when it does change, it will make the person aware that the time for meditation is complete. Vigilant behaviors and a concern about time are unnecessary because the music frames the experience from beginning to end.

As individuals become more experienced in meditation, they may find they can meditate without listening to music. It may not be necessary for them to hear the music each time meditation is desired, provided they can "think through" the music and hear it in their mind. This is particularly useful when it is inconvenient or impossible to play the music (e.g., other people are in the room who may not wish to hear the music) or when a cassette or compact disc player is inaccessible. Thinking through a piece of music used in meditation can help individuals access the peace and tranquility experienced in this state of consciousness. Mentally playing the music provides structure, predictability, and security as it evokes pleasant feelings or memories and the comfort associated with them. Consequently, it can provide relief from stressful or unpleasant situations, such as insomnia or fear associated with pain during illness.

Returning from a Meditative State

Once the time for meditation is complete, an individual must return to full consciousness. The return to consciousness may be facilitated by music that stimulates consciousness through familiarity and predictability. A gradual change in music is usually best. Like waking from a deep sleep, this process requires time for physical and psychological adjustments. The music may gradually increase in tempo from slow to legato (smooth and connected) to progressively faster and more upbeat. Rhythms may be syncopated. The music may also employ lyrics that are spiritually significant to the individual.

The interval of time required to resume full consciousness varies among and within individuals, according to the depth of their meditative states. Deeper states of meditation and quicker entry into these states are possible as individuals acquire more experience and learn how best to program their music to enhance their experiences.

USING MUSIC IN HEALING

Out of the most profound pain in life can come opportunities to transcend it and regain trust and feel nurtured through healing. Some of the deepest emotional pain results from physical, sexual (particularly incest), and emotional abuse and neglect. These severe personal violations rob individuals of their abilities to trust and to experience emotions other than fear and anxiety (O'Konski, 1994). Deep emotional pain also results from loss, such as the end of relationships through divorce or death, or from chronic disability, cultural changes, and regret. The grief associated with abuse, loss, and regret requires resolution (Bright, 1996). Psychological interventions may help identify and define the pain and can even offer insight into it, but healing comes only from spiritual experiences.

Healing is an active process that includes the following components: the experience of pain, identification of the pain and the cause, expression of pain, forgiveness, and resolution into well-being. The prerequisite to this process is the willingness to experience it. People who are unable to identify their pain and are unwilling to reveal their feelings must be allowed their privacy. To press them to delve into their past could be detrimental. Their need to express feelings or to engage in any aspect of grief work must come from them, not from professionals, clergy, friends, family members, or other so-called "helpers."

Healing begins with identifying and embracing the pain and understanding the void it creates (Arterburn, 2007). Numbing pain with denial, alcohol, drugs, or over-involvement in work, family, or social commitments only postpones healing. Pain is suppressed, perhaps for years, and surfaces only when the defenses against it are no longer practical. Many people who have suppressed or denied pain throughout their lifetime find themselves in later life heavily burdened by that pain. The following vignette illustrates the effects of numbing oneself to pain:

> Sister Sarah, a 70-year-old nun, had denied throughout her life a terrible experience she had as a child. She had never allowed herself to grieve over her experience, but bore her pain stoically. In a workshop conducted by a music therapist, she heard about using music to embrace pain. As the music therapist played some examples of music people could use, Sister Sarah began to sob uncontrollably. She ran from the workshop and spent several hours grieving over the event from her childhood. With support from workshop professional staff, Sister Sarah began her healing process.

The healing process resembles the process of peeling an onion. As one layer is grieved, subsequently healed, and peeled away, another layer is then revealed. The process of grieving, healing, and peeling continues until a state of well-being is achieved. Music may be used to access the pain and the feelings about it that have been denied. The use of music may begin with instrumental pieces that are preferred and selected by individuals. Preferred music is usually familiar music, and because it is part of an individuals' experience, it maintains associations with those experiences. Some of the associations may be with events that were significant in the individual's life. Although the feelings associated with the events may not be clear, individuals may be able to recall particular events and behaviors that the music brings to mind.

When the feelings are not clear, music should be selected with lyrics that reflect emotions associated with certain events or behaviors. Characteristically, lyrics are combined with musical elements that reflect emotions through melody, tonality, timbre, harmony, and rhythm. Inherent in this music is the understanding of emotions that composers and performers communicate. Often, people will say, "It was as if he was singing just to me. That song is my life story." This connection makes the music even more poignant and enhances opportunities for listeners to begin to access their emotions, at the least. Perhaps the music will also allow listeners to feel emotions for the first time. Results of a research study intended to determine the effects of music and spiritual beliefs on individuals' coping with emotional issues indicated that individuals' experiences with music helped them identify their long-buried feelings. Additionally, the study indicated that individuals could recognize song lyrics as an articulation of their feelings, and participants realized that they were not alone in their pain and frustration and understood that their feelings were valid (Pitts & Gierhart, 1995).

When people become aware of their emotions, it is important that they have someone with whom to discuss these emotions, to provide support as the emotions evolve, and to validate feelings as they surface. It is also important to allow the feelings to unfold at whatever rate the person can tolerate. Some people may need to recognize feelings and then briefly step back from them in order to adjust to a certain level of pain. They may return to continue the experience, but it must happen in their own time and at a level that they can tolerate.

At least at first, pain may be difficult to access for people who have denied their feelings all their lives for fear of reprisal, disapproval, or abuse. These people most likely did not experience open emotional expression in their families, and they learned early in their lives that such expressions were unacceptable (Bradshaw, 2005). Although these people may verbalize a desire to express themselves, they do not know how to do so because they did not have role models to imitate. Others know only that they are not happy and want something better. They are able to say that they feel deep unhappiness and remorse, but they do not know the cause. When asked to name their grief and the source of it, they may ask how they should structure their responses. They may ask, "What can I say? I don't even know who I am. How can I say what I feel? Can you tell me what to do or say to feel better?" They have little or no experience with feelings, let alone experience identifying and discussing any issues associated with them. It is essential to facilitate and support their efforts without making judgments.

Music can help people identify their feelings through associations with other people's experiences. Analyses of lyrics that describe feelings may provide some opportunities for clarification. Individuals may be asked to determine whether a lyric directly reflects something about how they feel. They may simply agree or disagree. They may be asked to elaborate; however, they should do so only if they feel comfortable sharing further information. Care must be taken to not overwhelm individuals. Experiencing feelings may overwhelm them and deplete their energy to cope with daily functions. Often, it is best for individuals to cope with one feeling at a time. The feeling must identified by the individual as the most prominent and the one with which they wish to begin work.

Expressing Grief

Bright (1996) has indicated that expressions of grief are necessary for people to move into the future. Individuals must decide to commit themselves to the effort. The amount and type of self-expression they require depends on their perception of the amount of damage they have suffered. One incident, such as the death of a spouse, may be perceived as extremely painful by one person and as a relief by another person, who has experienced anticipatory grief during a prolonged chronic illness, such as cancer or Alzheimer's disease. Even with this preliminary grief work, a sense of loss occurs with death and may bring with it a new set of issues, such as regrets associated with decisions and events earlier in life. "If only" thoughts may surface. For instance, "*If only* I had married my first sweetheart, I would have better financial circumstances." "*If only* I had gotten the diagnosis earlier, maybe my wife would still be alive." "*If only* I had worked harder at providing care, maybe we would have had more quality time." Other people may say that they are sad yet confident that their life was as good as it could have been, but now life has changed. Whatever the situation, the expression of pain leads to eventual acceptance.

Grief is manifested through various forms, such as tears, gestures, and verbalizations (e.g., talking with others, talking to oneself, singing). Recording thoughts and feelings in a journal or diary, writing poetry, and composing songs are other ways to grieve. When it is not possible to express grief in words, vocalizations can be helpful. The beginning of this expression is a sound that is more like a groan or a grunt. Individuals may be self-conscious and reluctant to express themselves in this way, although it may be the only form of expression they are able to access. Background music can support their efforts by masking these sounds and by providing them with some support and structure as they express their pain. The type of background music can vary in effect, depending on individuals' musical preferences. The author has found that bagpipe music has some important characteristics that promote vocalization. First, the music is centered around a droning tone, a sound that remains on one pitch. A vocal sound can match the pitch, but if it does not, it still fits naturally within the context of the music. Second, the music has a slow march-like tempo without accented beats, which provides a feeling of structure without strong stimulation for physical movement. Therefore, the music is compatible with continuous vocal sounds that can increase in volume as individuals become more comfortable within the structure of the music. Third, the sound of the music is continuous for the duration of a selection. This continuity allows individuals to vocalize, take a breath when needed, and vocalize again.

As people vocalize along with music, they become increasingly engaged in their feelings. It is as if the vocalizations trigger individuals' awareness of their emotions. They may cry, wail, and even scream in their grief and must be encouraged to do so. If individuals are concerned about others hearing them, they can be advised to find a place where they can be alone. They may cry or scream into a pillow or mattress, but it must be done so with abandon to trigger the healing process.

Forgiving

Forgiveness is an essential step in healing, but it is ineffective without an awareness of what precipitated the need to heal (Levine, 1991). The reason(s) for the pain, the events that surrounded the pain, and grief over the pain are prerequisites to forgiveness. The pain may result from others' actions, but it also may be a consequence of one's own behavior. It may stem from someone else's wrongdoing or it may result from regret. In such a case, there is a need for self-forgiveness. Some pain may result from events that were beyond one's control, such as a fatal illness, death, or other emotional or physical trauma. In these cases, there is a need to forgive God.

Initially, forgiveness is not a feeling, but an act of will that requires practice. It is done not once but repeatedly. Forgiving finishes the business of grieving, but in forgiving, one does not condone the actions that precipitated it (Levine, 1991). To end grief, it is necessary to forgive. Forgiveness is part of spiritually letting go. Through forgiveness, there is access to spiritual recovery, no matter how terrible the hurt. Although the words "I forgive" may not come easily, they begin the process of personal acknowledgment and the desire for spiritual intervention in the healing process. When one forgives, one may also say things like "I hurt," "It is truly awful; I don't know if I can even live through this," or "I forgive because I want to be happy again."

Statements of forgiveness may be incorporated into chants. These chants provide a structure for behaviors that are difficult to implement because the feelings of pain are still strong and not naturally compatible with feelings of forgiveness. Initially, these chants may seem forced, but eventually the chanting becomes less an expression of anger and hurt and more an expression of acceptance and relinquished control. The quality of the voice, therefore, is a reflection of the emotions of the individual.

In addition to chanting, individuals may use music to establish an environment for physical relaxation, which represents another form of relinquishing control. Music that evokes feelings of comfort and calm must be selected in this context. Individuals may choose to listen while either sitting or reclining. They must not be interrupted or distracted. A progressive muscle relaxation technique or an autogenic (produced independent of external influences or aid) approach may be used. Individuals may then spend some time focusing on their breathing while listening to their music. They may think of breathing in forgiveness and breathing out pain, suffering, and ugliness. After some time, they may release their focus and allow the music to relax them until the end of the selection. This approach can be practiced several times a day.

Resolving Grief

Relief from pain and grief evolves over time. Relief is fleeting at first. There may be only a moment when pain is not experienced. That one moment may be the only time during a day that one does not spend suffering, but it is nonetheless a beginning. As forgiveness occurs, these moments become more frequent. During this part of the healing process, people may need to rest from the hard work of healing in order to enjoy the amount of recovery from pain and grief they have already experienced. Eventually, they will experience more time feeling happiness than pain.

The role of music in well-being lies in the association it has with feelings of peace, tranquility, and joy. Music can be used to evoke these positive feelings on a regular basis or whenever people feel a sense of insecurity or apprehension in dealing with painful issues. Whatever the case, music provides them with stability, security, and their associated comforts.

CONCLUSION

Spirituality is an individual experience that must be pursued alone. Although spirituality carries with it great responsibility, it brings great joy, calm, and a connection that exceeds human understanding (Peck, 2003). Music can be used to enhance or even provide spiritual experiences by establishing a context within which prayer or ritual can be conducted; by evoking emotional responses; and by awakening values, memories, and beliefs. It can also contribute to spirituality by removing distractions, directing attention, and providing security in solitude. All these characteristics of music can be used by individuals to help them on their spiritual journeys as they experience God.

REFERENCES

Arterburn, S. (2007). *Healing is a choice: 10 decisions that will transform your life and 10 lies that can prevent you from making them*. Nashville: Thomas Nelson.

Bradshaw, J. (2005). *Healing the shame that binds you* (Rev. ed). Deerfield Beach, FL: Health Communications.

Bright, R. (1996). *Grief and powerlessness: Helping people regain control of their lives*. London: Jessica Kingsley.

Campbell, J., & Fairchild, J. E. (1993). *Myths to live by*. New York: Penguin Books.

The cloud of unknowing. (1979). (W. Johnston, Trans.). New York: Doubleday. (Original work printed 14th century)

Dossey, L. (1997). *Healing words: The power of prayer and the practice of medicine* (New ed.). New York: HarperOne.

Fowler, J. (1995). *Stages of faith: The psychology of human development*. San Francisco: HarperOne.

Gaston, E. T. (1968). Man and music. In E. T. Gaston (Ed.), *Music in therapy* (pp. 7–29). New York: Macmillan Press.

Levine, S. (1991). *Guided meditation, explorations and healings* (2nd ed.). New York: Anchor Books.

Merriam, A. (1964). *Anthropology of music*. Chicago: Northwestern University Press.

Moore, T. (1992). *The care of the soul: A guide for cultivating depth and sacredness in everyday life*. New York: HarperPaperbacks.

Naranjo, C. (1979). *Meditation: Its spirit and techniques*. In C.

Naranjo & R. Ornstein (Eds.), On the psychology of meditation (pp. 2–132). New York: Viking Press.

O'Konski, M. (1994). *Rationale for music therapy in the treatment of individuals who experienced childhood sexual abuse.* Unpublished manuscript, University of Kansas, Lawrence.

Ornstein, R. (1979). The techniques of meditation and their implications for modern psychology. In C. Naranjo & R. Ornstein (Eds.), *On the psychology of meditation* (pp. 133–248). New York: Viking Press.

Peck, M. S. (2003). *The road less traveled* (25th anniversary ed.). New York: Touchstone.

Pitts, C. A., & Gierhart, L. (1995). *Affirming adult psychiatric patients spiritual beliefs as a coping mechanism using lyric analysis and song writings: A total quality management approach.* Unpublished manuscript, Colorado Mental Health Institute, Fort Logan.

Thaut, M. (2005). Neuropsychological processes in music perception and their relevance in music therapy. In R. F. Unkefer & M. H. Thaut (Eds.), *Music therapy in the treatment of adults with mental disorders* (pp. 2–32). Gilsum, NH: Barcelona.

Chapter 10

Using Music to Help the Caregiver

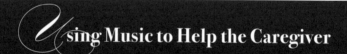

Using Music to Help the Caregiver

Caregivers need education and support to ensure high quality caregiving. Whether the caregivers are spouses, family members, or professionals, their education is generally focused on the benefits of certain interventions for the care recipient. Some education is available concerning the maintenance of caregivers' physical and emotional health through good nutrition, exercise, stress management, proper rest, and the pursuit of interests for self-stimulation outside their caregiver role. This information is available through literature, workshops, support groups, and professional training. However, there has been a failure to provide information on ways caregivers can cope with their own emotional reactions, maintain emotional intimacy, promote a sense of belonging to family for the people for whom they care, and promote good quality in their own relationships.

Music can provide opportunities for spouse and family caregivers to share something that goes beyond the fulfillment of day-to-day physical needs with the people for whom they provide care. Music can enhance interactions (verbal or nonverbal), trigger memories, promote feelings of closeness, and create an opportunity for emotional intimacy between caregivers and care recipients.

CARING FOR CAREGIVERS OF PEOPLE WITH DEMENTIA

People with dementia require an increasing amount of care as their disease progresses. Research shows that family caregivers experience emotional reactions associated with the diagnosis of dementia; a deep sense of loss as the disease progresses (Barnes, Raskind, Scott, & Murphy, 1981; Papastavrou, Kalokerinou, Papacostas, Tsangari, & Sourtzi, 2007); depression (Meyers & Alexopoulos, 1988; Tanji et al., 2005); and loneliness as they lose the companionship of a loved one, experience social isolation and increased responsibility, and suffer emotional burdens that seriously affect their quality of life (Bergman-Evans, 1994; Rose-Rego, Strauss, & Smyth, 1998).

With each stage of progressive dementia come specific needs, issues, and problems that affect both the caregiver and the care recipient. As functioning is lost by the recipient of care, the caregiver's responsibilities and burdens of providing care grow. These responsibilities and burdens are difficult to cope with, particularly when the relationship between the caregiver and the care recipient was unsatisfying before the onset of illness. A woman related the distress she felt concerning the care she was providing for her husband of 42 years when she was asked to participate in a couples' music therapy group with him:

> My husband and I have always had a difficult time. He is my second husband, and when I married him my daughter was 6 years old. Things were rocky from the start. He was gruff with my little girl and slapped her around a lot. Whenever I tried to intervene, he popped me good. I can't tell you how many black eyes and other bruises he gave me. Now, after years and years of taking his abuse, I have to take care of him. I really want all this to be over, but I know that I have to endure. I just really resent all the time and energy he takes from me, and I really don't want to be a part of a group with him.

The pathology of the husband's dementia added to the misery that had always been a part of this couple's relationship. This woman expressed no interest in having any interaction with her husband outside of the care she felt obligated to provide at home. For her, techniques for stress management and expressions of anger were much more appropriate.

Using Music in Early-Stage Dementia

People with early-stage dementia are most likely able to attend to their own personal care. They are able to continue to socialize with familiar people and appear normal to people who do not know them. However, their emotions tend to flatten and they begin to withdraw from activities that are unfamiliar or may present a challenge (Reisberg, Ferris, Leon, & Crook, 1982). The caregiver's role in early-stage dementia could include helping with finances, arranging transportation and other activities that are unfamiliar, and providing emotional support.

Although they are not required to supervise daily tasks and the moment-to-moment activities of loved ones with early-stage dementia, family members are faced with the deterioration that is to come. They may have difficulty accepting this inevitability and may deny the facts, at least for a time. They may try to make excuses for their loved one, but as behaviors fit increasingly into the model of degenerative dementia, they begin to accept the inevitable.

Acceptance of dementia brings grief and disappointment to family caregivers, and dreams for the future die. Often, family members (spouses included) report that they did not plan for things to turn out the way that they did. They believed that they would have time to enjoy travel, mutual interests, family visits, and other activities with their loved ones. However, dementia robbed them of that time.

As caregivers work through the grief process, they may feel angry. They have periods of deep sadness and great distress. These feelings are also felt by their care recipients. Consequently, caregivers must cope not only with their own emotional reactions to the disease, but with those of their loved ones as well.

Support groups are available for people with early-stage dementia and their caregivers, but it may not be enough just to talk with others about grief and frustration. Caregivers and care recipients need to nonverbally express the feelings associated with having an untreatable, incurable disease. They also need to experience relief from the reality of progressive dementia. To do so, caregivers must define and use skills and strengths that can provide them with some satisfaction in life. Simply stated, they must take time just for themselves.

For many people with early-stage dementia who participated in music before onset of the disease, music evokes feelings of success and satisfaction when other less familiar activities evoke feelings of failure and dissatisfaction. Making music together provides caregivers and their care recipients with some power over conditions that are beyond their control. Making music taps skills that are still intact and abilities that allow opportunities for meaningful engagement with loved ones. Music allows caregivers and care recipients to interact without the pain of loss. Caregivers can use these experiences to help them focus on the strengths and residual abilities of their loved ones and leave behind, albeit briefly, their fear and apprehension of what is to come.

Successful participation in music offers delightful musical interactions between caregivers and care recipients without the attendant sadness of disease and loss, as in the following vignette:

A daughter who had often played piano duets with her mother continued to do so after her mother was diagnosed with dementia. The music they had always played together remained familiar to the mother and she could still play it well. As they played together, their positive experiences of sharing music allowed them to enjoy the music and each other and to forget their distress. The daughter knew that her mother would eventually lose the ability to play music with her and she wanted to cherish whatever positive experiences remained.

People who have not performed music with others during their adult lives may share music they have in common in other ways. Caregivers may ask their loved ones with dementia to sing songs with them that they both know—perhaps songs that mothers or fathers sang to them when they were children; songs that couples sang or danced to in their early years together; or songs that were common at home, school, or church. Sharing this music provides a nonthreatening way for caregivers to interact with their loved ones with dementia. Thus, care recipients' participation in music becomes a resource for caregivers. Caregivers can use care recipients' participation to ensure success, especially when their loved ones with dementia feel discouraged and unsettled. Participation can also help their loved ones find alternatives to distressing experiences and offer opportunities for loved ones to retain some control.

Away from their loved ones with dementia, caregivers may express their deep feelings of pain and hurt through singing. The singing may sound more like groaning. This groaning may be the initial vocalization that leads to verbal expressions of anger and grief. With these initial vocalizations, caregivers can begin to put their feelings into words. As caregivers continue to label and express their feelings through words, they may begin to write poetry that can be set to music, or they may rewrite lyrics of existing songs. Whatever form music composition takes, it is a helpful and useful way for caregivers to express their innermost feelings about the dementia of a loved one. Caregivers can also express their feelings by playing an instrument. Music lessons can provide an opportunity for enjoyable personal development for caregivers who have never played an instrument.

If caregivers do not wish to make music, they may wish to

study music history, with a focus on their family's culture or some other context. Part of this study can include listening to music and visiting the local library, because books and recordings can provide enjoyable outings for both caregivers and their care recipients.

Listening to music can also enhance caregivers' quality of life by helping to manage their stress. When combined with relaxation techniques (see Appendices A, B, and C), these musical interludes in the daily routine provide mini-vacations from caregiving duties. By using music and relaxation for 20–30 minutes each morning and afternoon, people can receive temporary respite from worry and fear.

Using Music in Middle-Stage Dementia

As dementia progresses into the middle stage and further cognitive ability is lost, it places further demands on caregivers. They do the best that they can, often making excuses for the care recipient in the community. Caregivers may also make excuses for themselves. If invited to a social function, caregivers may excuse themselves by explaining that they are not feeling well, that their rheumatism is acting up, that their gallbladder is causing them trouble, that they already have plans with their new grandchild, or that they are simply too busy.

Caregivers may hold onto the facade they constructed in the early stages of the dementia that everything is fine until the care recipient's behavior deteriorates to the extent that it is impossible to continue doing so (e.g., leaving the house in the middle of the night dressed inadequately and resisting returning home when found; resorting to crying or throwing tantrums in a public place in response to frustration or fear; wandering away from the caregiver during a routine shopping excursion, resulting in a need to call the police). Such displays of behaviors make members of the community aware of the loved one's dementia. Often, caregivers respond by isolating themselves further. Although caregivers may be somewhat relieved that their situation is known, they may continue to avoid contact with others.

Caregivers sacrifice their own needs to provide for their loved ones with dementia. They tolerate behaviors that make them uncomfortable in order to avoid confrontations that may have catastrophic results. They also make every effort to promote calm and tranquility. Mrs. Bando explains the behaviors she tolerates from her husband:

> My Dan was always good with his hands. He could fix just about anything, and he did all the maintenance on our car. He once rebuilt an engine of an old pickup truck we purchased that didn't run well enough to suit him. With his dementia, though, he has quit working on engines, but he leaves his tools all over the house. I find them on the coffee table, on the dresser in the bedroom, and in the bathroom sink. If I ask him to put them away, he gets upset and tells me that he needs his tools because he has things to do. I guess leaving his tools all over the house isn't so bad. I once had to use a pair of pliers to turn the water off and on in the kitchen sink when he took the handles off and I couldn't find them. Eventually I found them at the bottom of his sock drawer.

Taking time out for themselves is essential for caregivers like Mrs. Bando. Using relaxation techniques while listening to music (see Appendices A, B, and C) is an important way to release tension and manage stress. Another important technique is affirmations, which help caregivers to remember their worth. Affirmation is a process of repeating statements to oneself that describe the self positively while breathing rhythmically. Such statements include "I am a good person," "I am worthwhile," "I am loved," "I am filled with kindness," "I am fine just the way I am," "I do the best I can," and "I am the best me I can be." These affirmations are important for self-encouragement and self-acceptance, especially when the care recipient provides no affirming verbal feedback. Affirmations can be accompanied by music that is special and meaningful to provide a brief diversion from the demands of the day.

Just as familiar music serves care recipients in their needs for comfort and relief from stress, familiar music is important for caregivers, who find that each day has unpredictable, equilibrium-disturbing situations involving the people to whom they provide care. When coping with care recipients with middle-stage dementia, caregivers may use music to provide structure for nonverbal interactions with care recipients. Caregivers still need emotional feedback from the people in middle-stage dementia for whom they care, and when they do not receive it, they develop deep emotional deficits. Dance tunes from the big band era may be used to encourage care recipients to move in rhythm while they hold their caregivers in their arms (Clair, 2002). If dancing is not desirable, care recipients can sit opposite or by the side of their caregivers and hold them. The music provides a context for the physical contact involved in rocking back and forth together and leaning on one another's cheeks. Music encourages care recipients who are otherwise unable to focus their attention on loving, physical gestures to touch their caregivers. These loving gestures with musical background provide moments of emotional intimacy between caregivers and care recipients and significantly contribute to fulfilling caregivers' emotional needs.

Using Music in Late-Stage Dementia

When it becomes impossible to provide care at home, caregivers often resort to residential placement. Often, such placement is made only when the caregiver has developed or is likely to develop a serious illness or suffer physical injury in efforts to provide care at home. Caregivers often feel pressured to consider residential care for their loved ones, and they suffer emotional trauma as a result, even when circumstances are beyond their control. They reluctantly admit their inability to cope, and they express feelings of failure and regret that they were forced to "give up." They feel helpless, perhaps for the first time in their lives.

Mrs. Prather described feeling enormous guilt when she placed her husband of 42 years in a long-term care facility:

> My Ben is the sweetest guy. We have just had a wonderful marriage, the second for both of us. I had a miserable time before we met and so did he. We hit it off and decided that we could have a happy life together, and indeed, we have. It just breaks my heart that it has ended up this way.
>
> I kept Ben at home for as long as I could after he was diagnosed with progressive dementia. He is a very large man and has always been very determined to have his way. He's always

been so protective of me. As he suffered more and more memory losses, I found I could no longer manage his behaviors to take care of his physical needs. He fought me when I tried to change his soiled clothes, he physically pushed me away when I tried to help him bathe, and because he napped through the day, he wandered through the house all night, unable to sleep. After I reached a point of exhaustion, my son insisted that I put him in nursing care. I felt so very bad about what I had to do, but I hadn't slept through the night in 2 years and I was at the end of my rope.

After I put Ben in the care home, I lay awake each night wondering if maybe I hadn't tried hard enough. Maybe I could've handled him a while longer. I just couldn't reconcile giving up until my friends convinced me that I had to take care of myself, so I could continue to take care of Ben. After some weeks of visiting him every day, I could see that he got the kind of care I couldn't give him at home. I went to several of the support group meetings, and I began to see that I wasn't the only one who felt this way.

My son and my friends have been awfully good to me. I am so glad to have my husband in such good hands. I know it's the best thing for him, and for me, too.

Unlike Mrs. Prather, some caregivers cannot admit that they can no longer cope, and they place their loved ones in residential care for respite with the intention of taking their loved one home with them once they recover from their exhaustion or illness and feel capable of giving care once again. Sometimes the relief from the burdens of caregiving is so great that caregivers eventually indicate a desire to permanently place their loved ones in residential care. This decision is not an easy one by any means and often requires support from friends, family, and residential care staff.

Other caregivers accept the inevitability of full-time residential placement, but make every effort to postpone it as long as possible. They postpone placement in order to maintain their own health and well-being. With support and encouragement, they are willing to indulge their own needs for a while. They may schedule respite care in a residential facility for their loved one for several days or weeks in order to take a vacation, to visit family, to clean the house, or to enjoy the peace and tranquility of being at home alone. Some caregivers use adult day services, which provide them with opportunities to care for themselves, do household chores, shop for groceries, and participate in community activities while their loved ones are away for the day. In addition, caregivers may schedule home health care services for their loved ones, provided they qualify for the services. Home health aides perform tasks that are beyond caregivers' capabilities but are necessary to the health and quality of life of the care recipient.

In the later stage of dementia, loved ones with the disease can no longer carry on meaningful conversations with their caregivers, but caregivers still need some type of interaction with their loved ones. They may continue to visit their loved ones regularly, but often leave the facility disappointed and saddened by their inability to engage them in meaningful interactions. Hope Renfrew, a caregiving daughter, described her visits with her father as follows:

> My dad was a surgeon who led quite an exciting life. He used to garden for relaxation and grew some of the most gorgeous roses in the city. When I come to visit Dad here at the care home, I take him out on the garden walk, and I try to get him to look at the plantings with me. I stop to look, but he just continues to shuffle on his way. He seems oblivious to me or to the plants that he once enjoyed so much. I really don't know what to do with him, so I just walk with him until he gets tired and heads for the door to go inside. He always loved music, too. He often would sit and listen to it while he read for very long periods of time. Now he can only sit for 4 or 5 minutes before he gets up to wander.

A model music therapy program was tested with couples (spouses and adult children and their parents), in which one member of the couple was the caregiver and the other had late-stage dementia, to open opportunities for interaction to people like Hope Renfrew and her father. All care recipients were in residential care and had lost their ability to carry on meaningful conversations. The care recipients were still ambulatory, but were not purposeful in their behaviors. The study group consisted of three or four couples who met in two weekly sessions of 50 minutes each. Each session began with 10 minutes of conversation among the caregivers, progressed to 10 minutes of singing, 10 minutes of ballroom dancing, and 10 minutes of drum playing. The sessions concluded with 10 minutes of conversation among the caregivers. The results showed that couples participated well together using ballroom dancing and drumming but, although caregivers enjoyed talking with one another and singing together, they noted that the care recipients participated only minimally. Care recipients did some singing, but generally were not able to join in the conversations (Clair & Ebberts, 1997). When asked to evaluate the contributions music therapy made to their visits, caregivers reported that music therapy gave structure to their participation. They said that in their previous visits they were unable to elicit responses from their loved ones. Some caregivers said that they were frustrated by and disappointed in their earlier visits, but that they felt too guilty to stay away. Consequently, they came regularly to see their loved ones, only to have nothing to do when they were with them except follow them around as they wandered or sit with them, unable to converse. The caregivers indicated that they derived a great deal of satisfaction from interacting with their loved ones using music.

In a later study, a family caregiver was taught to carry out a musical engagement with a loved one. The music therapist introduced singing, playing drums, and ballroom dancing as the choices to each caregiver who brought his or her loved one to the session. Caregivers chose one of the three music activities and the music therapist helped facilitate for the first two weekly sessions. In four subsequent sessions caregivers implemented the chosen musical activity independently while the music therapist observed. All caregivers commented that they felt competent and confident to carry on the music-centered visits independently after the series of six sessions ended (Clair, 2002). It was clear that family caregivers were capable of learning and implementing music activities as a way to engage their care receivers and that they were quite successful and satisfied with their efforts.

When individuals become so debilitated by the disease process that they are no longer ambulatory, family members can continue to make contact with them using music. For example, they may sing songs well known to care recipients because they heard their mother sing the songs to them or they memorized them as youths at school or church. The musical selection is best determined by family members, who know the history of the care recipients and who wish to use song to elicit some response from them.

Often, care recipients in late-stage dementia respond to the singing of the loved ones by making eye contact or by vocalizing at particular points in a song. The following vignettes illustrate the effect singing can have on care recipients and their caregivers:

> Mr. Crenshaw had been in residential care for several years. During music therapy, he always responded to a phrase in the song "God Bless America," by Irving Berlin. A veteran of World War II, Mr. Crenshaw cried out each time the lyric "God bless America, my home sweet home" was sung. His response seemed purposeful because it was made in the same way with the same facial expression every time the phrase was sung. It seemed as though he was singing along.

> Mrs. Stanislawski was visiting her husband while he was hospitalized for pneumonia. She wanted to interact with him, even though he had been mute for over 3 years. Encouraged by a music therapist to sing her husband's favorite song, Mrs. Stanislawski used some of their time alone to sing to him. She reported that when her husband heard her sing, he held her gaze and his face had a familiar expression. She said that she knew she had made contact that was no longer possible otherwise, and that she felt connected to him. Mr. Stanislawski died unexpectedly some weeks later. Mrs. Stanislawski told the music therapist that she would always remember the peaceful, serene look on his face each time she sang to him, and she thanked the music therapist for this gift, something she would cherish for the rest of her life.

> Mrs. Ostvald observed a music therapist working with her husband, who was in residential care. She commented to the therapist that she enjoyed watching him respond to singing. Mrs. Ostvald was encouraged to sing to her husband, and af-

ter numerous attempts to persuade her, she agreed. Meeting with the music therapist, Mrs. Ostvald said that she missed getting close to her husband and hugging him. The music therapist suggested that she sit with him in his hospital bed while she sang. Mrs. Ostvald gasped at the suggestion. "Do you think it would be all right?" she asked. The music therapist said it would be fine. As the therapist left, Mrs. Ostvald took off her shoes, climbed into bed to sit beside her husband, crossed her ankles, put her arm around him, and sang "You Are My Sunshine" while he gazed into her eyes.

PRESERVING PRICELESS MEMORIES

When satisfying experiences occur with music, it is important to preserve them so they can be reviewed at a later time. One way to preserve these experiences is to video record them. Lois Johnson Morelock, who provided care to her husband until he died from probable Alzheimer's disease, counsels families to record their positive experiences with their loved ones with dementia while they can still interact. She suggests using music to sing together, and when that is no longer possible, to continue dancing together for as long as possible.

As she counsels families, Mrs. Morelock teaches them about the progression of dementia, but emphasizes the maintenance of abilities that are possible using music. Videos capture memories of happier and better times, especially in the later stages of the disease process when care recipients no longer respond to family members. Morelock stresses that the care recipient is a person who has an identity as an important family member, even after dementia strips everything away. Morelock has found the videos of her husband's successful participations in music therapy to be a source of comfort, especially following his death. His disease process was long and painful for her and her children. Using the videos has reminded them of some good times, memories that push all the pain and distress into the background for a while and give them positive thoughts of the man who was a loving husband and father.

CAREGIVERS OF PEOPLE IN PALLIATIVE CARE

As they age, people may develop illnesses that require skilled nursing care. These ailments are often long-lasting and recovery may not be possible. The effort to keep these people comfortable, with no pain or physical distress, and to diminish their emotional suffering can be met through palliative care. In many cases, however, little is done for the spouse or other family member who has responsibility for their care. Often, caregiving spouses are older and frail themselves, and visiting their loved ones challenges their health and well-being . Simply traveling to visit may be difficult. If the caregiver no longer drives or never drove a car, other transportation must be arranged. This may present problems. For example, moving quickly enough to get on and off trains or buses and navigating steps and/or escalators to enter and exit mass transit systems can be difficult for older people or people with disabilities. Travel by taxi may be an option, but is beyond the financial means of many people.

After coping with the difficulties of transportation, caregivers may be disheartened further when faced with the condition of their loved ones. Residents of nursing facilities may be forlorn and depressed because there has been little or no improvement in their condition. Caregivers know they are there to bring hope and encouragement to their loved ones, but they may be barely able to muster these emotions. They approach their visits in a spirit of giving, but with limited or no resources to draw on, they can experience burnout. As their energy reserves are already diminished by their day-to-day struggles, they are depleted further by difficult confrontations with their ill and frail loved ones. With each encounter, caregivers may feel that they have less to contribute. They may become greatly fatigued and fall ill themselves. A young woman recounted the difficulties that her grandparents faced:

> I don't know what to do about my grandparents. My grandpa had a heart attack about 15 years ago. He had to retire because he just couldn't do his job anymore. He was a laborer all his life, and all he did was work. He was really lost, since he had nothing that interested him. He has no hobbies. He just filled his life with work from the time he woke up in the morning

until he went to bed at night. Then, about 7 years ago, his condition became so bad that my grandma couldn't take care of him anymore, and he went into the nursing home. Now, he just lies in bed all day, and he's getting more and more depressed. I really worry about my grandma. She's 87 years old and goes to visit him every day. She told me last week that Grandpa told her to get his gun because he just wanted to die. When I asked Grandma what she did about the gun, she said that she just ignored him, rubbed his back, and talked to him about us kids. When my grandma goes to visit him, she sits with him for 4 or 5 hours. She is there to feed him lunch and supper because he won't eat unless someone stays with him. I think about her sitting there all that time everyday. I don't know what to do to help her. I have to keep my job, and I'm 300 miles away.

Self-Care and Structuring Visits to Promote Caregiver Well-Being

The granddaughter in the previous case consulted a therapist for advice for her grandmother. The therapist made two suggestions: take care of herself (self-care) and structure her daily visits. Self-care includes stress management techniques that incorporate relaxation, physical maintenance through exercise, good nutrition, proper rest, the emotional support of family and friends, spiritual grounding (e.g., going to church or synagogue, praying, reading), and opportunities to pursue personal interests outside the caregiving role.

Self-care takes time, but it is critical for caregivers to maintain their physical and emotional well-being. Without attention to self-care, caregivers will suffer burnout. Caregivers may require assistance from their support system (e.g., family members, friends, volunteers from the community). A support system can make a significant contribution to a caregiver's health by substituting for the caregiver at scheduled times during the day. When several caregivers are involved in visiting the loved one, the visits can be organized around times that allow the primary caregiver to pursue various activities in the community (e.g., attendance at church services, participation in an exercise class, trips to the grocery store, cooking, opportunities to socialize with friends, relaxing).

Although daily visits are stressful, many caregivers feel they are necessary to honor feelings of loyalty and love in a relationship. Consequently, for these caregivers, making fewer visits is not an option as a stress reliever. Some other form of relief is required to alleviate stress during visits at nursing care facilities. Relief may come through incorporating some of the care recipients' interests into portions of the visits. When inquiries were made into the musical interests of the grandfather in the aforementioned case study, it was discovered that he had never listened to music. He was not fond of any particular type of music, but he was very proud of his grandchildren, who all happened to play musical instruments or sing. Because geographic proximity precluded frequent visits from his grandchildren to give live performances for their grandfather, they consented to make audio recordings their grandmother could play for him. The recordings included songs and instrumental music performed and dedicated especially to the grandfather. The recordings were further personalized by narration concerning the music (e.g., its history, its significance, who played on the original recording), along with a request for him to listen to it. The grandchildren made follow-up telephone calls to their grandfather to discuss the recorded music presentations.

The grandfather was receptive to listening to his grandchildren perform and to hearing some of their recordings each day. Although the grandchildren recorded and sent him new music periodically, he never tired of listening to all of their performances. The recordings seemed to lift his spirits, which improved the condition of the visits for his wife and alleviated her stress. She no longer felt the need to be with him every moment because he could play the music himself. She and her husband could share the music, which led to conversations about their children, grandchildren, and family events throughout their life together. The music recordings also provoked discussion when family and friends came to visit. Often the grandfather asked visitors to listen to his latest recording.

As the older couple in the previous case history discovered, music that is familiar to both caregivers and care recipients can fill and enhance the time they have together. Caregivers can let go of the responsibility they feel to maintain their loved ones' comfort by allowing the music to take over. Visiting loved ones can become a more positive experience as conversations about events or people associated with the music take the place of physical complaints. In addition, when the visit is over and the music is left behind to provide comfort, another burden of responsibility for caregivers is eased. When caregivers return home, they no longer feel as though they have abandoned their loved ones, but that they have left them in a positive environment.

Tactile Stimulation and Music

Music can be used in combination with other forms of sensory stimulation, such as massage. When caregivers need to communicate their feelings of love, combat their feelings of helplessness, and do something purposeful for their loved ones, they may find massage useful. Tactile stimulation conveys feelings of love and support (Edvardsson, Sandman, & Rasmussen, 2003; Skovdahl, Sörlie, & Kihlgren, 2007; Snyder, 1985) and can be used by caregivers to communicate feelings nonverbally to their loved ones. There is some indication that touching the back and lower arms in particular expresses understanding and sympathy (Pratt & Mason, 1984).

People can be massaged either by deeply rubbing and manipulating the muscles with rhythmic motions, or by lightly and rhythmically brushing with the fingers on the back from the shoulders down to the waist, on the legs from the knees to the ankles, on the feet from the heels to the toes, or on the arms from the shoulders to the fingertips. When coupled with music, the motions of massage are matched to the rhythm to help care recipients to relax (see Appendices A, B, and C), to facilitate communication of feelings, and to distract care recipients from their discomforts. The multi-sensory stimulation of touch and sound can also raise a person's awareness and may elicit responses from people who are generally unresponsive.

The therapeutic benefits of music and massage are facilitated if the music is familiar and enjoyed by care recipients and is compatible with caregivers' musical tastes (e.g., music danced to by a care recipient with dementia and her care-giving spouse). This music evokes positive memories and associations and provides an enjoyable and familiar context for touching. The following vignette is an example of how music and massage helped a grandfather and granddaughter reestablish their connection.

Mr. Jakot, 82, had a stroke and was admitted to the local medical center for acute care and rehabilitation. Although he had been hospitalized for a number of weeks, he did not seem to be getting any better. Any attempts on the part of his daughter and granddaughter to intervene were thwarted by Mr. Jakot's hearing loss. In addition, his vision was seriously impaired and he could not identify people standing next to him unless he could hear them speak. His granddaughter expressed her concern to a music therapist in the following way:

"I really think my granddad has given up. I go to see him in the hospital and he just lies there. When I try to talk to him, he doesn't seem able to hear me. I have to stand over him and yell in his ear for him to respond at all to me. I feel like he's shutting me out, and I have always been close to him. He is very important in my life, and I just can't stand to see him like this. Is there anything I can do with music to help? At least maybe I would feel like I was doing something."

After investigating further, the music therapist discovered that Mr. Jakot enjoyed watching "The Lawrence Welk Show" on television and his granddaughter often sat with him during the program. He could see little of the television picture, but he could hear the music by using special earphones to provide amplification.

The music therapist suggested to Mr. Jakot's granddaughter that she find recorded music by Lawrence Welk or other bands of the 1930s and 1940s and use a portable player with a headset on which to play the recordings at a volume her grandfather could hear. The therapist also suggested that she touch her grandfather to make him aware of her presence because his sight was so poor. In addition, she should tap his hand or shoulder in time to the dance music to stimulate the senses dulled by the stroke and to provide them both with loving contact.

CAREGIVERS OF PEOPLE IN INTENSIVE CARE

Caregivers are essential to the recovery process of severely ill or injured people that require intensive care to save their lives. It is also critical that the needs of caregivers are met in order for them to be with the patient whenever possible, to contribute to their care in some way, and to maintain their own health and well-being as they provide care (Dyer, 1991).

As treatment is focused on the patient's recovery, caregivers are generally left alone to cope with their distress. They may not sleep, eat, or rest well, and without the energy or the resources to care for themselves, they are at great risk for physical illness and emotional instability. Consequently, there is a need to intervene in order to prevent caregiver burnout.

Stress can be managed by using relaxation techniques with music. However, caregivers who are in shock over the serious illness or injury of a loved one may need others to help them with self-care, to use relaxation techniques with them, to sit with them, and to maintain their vigils for them at the hospital while they take some time to sleep. Nursing staff may also find it useful to have on hand some simple relaxation training techniques. Some intensive care units may make available players to families with selections of sedative music along with simple written instructions for relaxation. The most structured approach to relaxation will likely be the most productive for caregivers who are preoccupied with their loved one's distress, particularly if they have no previous experience with relaxation exercises. The muscle tense and release approach to relaxation found in Appendix A can serve as the basis for the written instructions. In addition, the relaxed jaw technique found in Appendix D is useful for caregivers who are unfamiliar with relaxation exercises.

Family members can be instructed to practice the relaxation exercises between visits to manage their stress. They may also be instructed to listen to familiar, comforting music before and after performing their relaxation exercises to control their stress further. Whatever comfort they can achieve by listening to music will not only add to their own well-being, but will be obvious to their loved ones during their visits. When patients in the intensive care unit are assured that loved ones are well, their attention can be focused on the healing process and not on the worry over the welfare of family members.

Caregivers can also make musical selections that can be used in their loved ones' care. This music can distract patients from their discomfort and can provide the family a role to play in the caregiving process. In addition, it is a way for family members to touch the patient, although physical contact may not be possible if injuries (e.g., burns) are extensive.

Playing music for patients in the intensive care unit can surround them with love and caring and the awareness that family members are with them in spirit, even when they are not physically present. At the same time, music allows family members to extend their touch and to provide contact through music that represents their feelings and thoughts. Music can facilitate patients' recovery and can maintain caregivers' well-being throughout the recovery process.

Conclusion

Music can provide an experience that caregivers and the people for whom they care can share. It can prompt reminiscence in people with dementia who can still converse meaningfully, it can give security and familiarity to a disorganized or institutional environment, and it can contribute a feeling of belonging to something, such as a family. When feelings of love and appreciation are no longer communicated verbally, music can help people to share them nonverbally.

REFERENCES

Barnes, R. F., Raskind, M. A., Scott, M., & Murphy, C. (1981). Problems of families caring for Alzheimer's patients: Use of a support group. *Journal of the American Geriatrics Society*, 29(2), 80–85.

Bergman-Evans, B. (1994). Alzheimer's and related disorders: Loneliness, depression, and social support of spousal caregivers. *Journal of Gerontological Nursing*, 20(3), 6–16.

Clair, A. A. (2002). The effects of music therapy on engagement in family caregiver and care receiver couples with dementia. *American Journal of Alzheimer's Disease and Other Dementias*, 17(5), 286–290.

Clair, A. A., & Ebberts, A. G. (1997). The effects of music therapy on interactions between family caregivers and their care receivers with late stage dementia. *Journal of Music Therapy*, 34(3), 148–164.

Dyer, I. (1991). Meeting the needs of visitors—A practical approach. *Intensive Care Nursing*, 7(3), 135–147.

Edvardsson, D. J., Sandman, P. O., & Rasmussen, B. H. (2003). Meaning of giving touch in the care of older patients: Becoming a valuable person and professional. *Journal of Clinical Nursing*, 12(4), 601–609.

Meyers, B. S., & Alexopoulos, G. S. (1988). Geriatric depression. *Medical Clinics of North America*, 72(4), 847–866.

Papastavrou, E., Kalokerinou, A., Papacostas, S. S., Tsangari, H., & Sourtzi, P. (2007). Caring for a relative with dementia: Family caregiver burden. *Journal of Advanced Nursing*, 58(5), 446–457.

Pratt, J., & Mason, A. (1984). The meaning of touch in care practice.

Social Science & Medicine, 18(12), 1081–1088.

Reisberg, B., Ferris, S. H., Leon, M. T, & Crook, T. (1982). The Global Deterioration Scale for assessment of primary degenerative dementia. *American Journal of Psychiatry*, 139(9), 1136–1139.

Rose-Rego, S. K., Strauss, M. E., Smyth, K. A. (1998). Differences in the perceived well-being of wives and husbands caring for persons with Alzheimer's disease. *The Gerontologist*, 38(2), 224–230.

Skovdahl, K., Sörlie, V., & Kihlgren, M. (2007). Tactile stimulation associated with nursing care to individuals with dementia showing aggressive or restless tendencies: An intervention study in dementia care. *International Journal of Older People Nursing*, 2(3), 162–170.

Snyder, M. (1985). *Independent nursing interventions*. New York: John Wiley & Sons.

Tanji, H., Ootsuki, M., Matsui, T., Maruyama, M., Nemoto, M., Tomita, N., Seki, T., Iwasaki, K., Arai, H., & Sasaki, H. (2005). Dementia caregivers' burdens and use of public services. *Geriatrics & Gerontology International*, 5(2), 94–98.

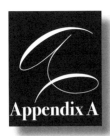

Appendix A

*P*rogressive Relaxation

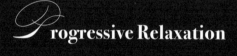

Progressive Relaxation

The progressive relaxation technique gradually relaxes muscles and brings calm to tense older people. The technique involves tightening, holding, and releasing a group of muscles and continuing this process in a sequence until all muscles in the body have been relaxed. Each muscle group is tightened, held, and released twice. More repetitions are possible, but fatigue may limit such activity. Do not "go for the burn." If any muscle groups still seem tight, repeat the relaxation technique.

The progressive relaxation technique must be conducted in a quiet room with subdued lighting, both of which facilitate relaxation. When providing instruction to the client, you should try to avoid the distraction of reading a script. Instead, record the instructions so you can play it as you work with the client. However, recorded instruction may present a problem depending on the type of electronic system with which you are working. In many cases, pacing cannot be adjusted to allow slower work with certain muscle groups, additional repetitions, or faster progression through certain exercises. If you do not have access to a system with remote control, or to simply allow for such adjustments, ask someone to provide instruction verbally as the exercises are performed. With practice and time it is generally possible to do the exercises from memory without listening to verbal instruction of any kind. Independence from external presentations of the script allows for individual differences and adjustments for particular tension in specific sets of muscles.

The progressive relaxation technique can be harmful in ways that include, but are not limited to, the following:

1. People with hypertension must not do the seven muscle groups or the four muscle groups techniques. Tensing large numbers of muscles simultaneously raises blood pressure and is strictly contraindicated for people with hypertension (Pender, Murdaugh, & Parsons, 2006).

2. Performing the relaxation technique may result in hypotension. Some people must remain seated for several minutes following total relaxation. Gradual movement should help the blood pressure to return to normal (Snyder, 1985). Taking such precautions means that the potential for dizziness and other symptoms of hypotension may be alleviated, and falls and injuries can be avoided.

3. People who have had myocardial infarction must not do the seven or the four muscle groups techniques, and they must not tense their muscles. Either activity will cause a large volume of blood to suddenly return to the heart. A damaged heart cannot handle sudden large volumes.

4. People who take medication and participate in relaxation should be carefully observed because trophotropic reactions, in which the responses of cells to nutritive substances are altered, can occur during relaxation. These reactions increase the potential effects of drugs and toxic levels may result. Trophotropic reactions may lead to hypoglycemia in people who take insulin and to overreactions to other medications. Lower dosage levels may be indicated in certain cases (Snyder, 1985).

5. The use of relaxation and visualization techniques should be avoided with people who have hallucinations or delusions because they may experience disturbances in reality as a result of relaxation or visualization (Snyder, 1985).

6. Depressed people may become increasingly withdrawn as they participate in relaxation and visualization techniques (Snyder, 1985). This reaction must be avoided.

7. People who tend to experience pervasive anxiety may respond to relaxation or visualization with heightened anxiety (e.g., exhibiting restlessness, breathing rapidly, shivering, perspiring profusely, trembling) (Heide & Borkovec, 1984). To avoid harmful reactions, do not use relaxation or visualization with anxious people.

8. People with chronic pain may find the relaxation and visualization techniques to be physically uncomfortable. For some people, it may increase their focus on pain and therefore may increase perceptions of it. If this response should occur, discontinue the relaxation or visualization technique (Snyder, 1985).

The scripts presented here may be used as provided or adjusted as desired. The sequence of muscle groups can be changed, and groups of muscles can be combined in order to progress more quickly through the sequence.

Music is helpful in performing the progressive relaxation

technique but is not always implemented. One reason may be that access to music is limited because of the setting in which the relaxation is performed (e.g., burn unit). Under such circumstances, music can be played mentally during the technique, provided practice has included music in active relaxation.

The musical selection must stimulate comfort and peace rather than a physical response, such as tapping the foot in rhythm. Sedate types of music that do not evoke physical responses are preferable, and these types of music must be individually selected because the effects of music are individually determined. In general, sedate music has a slow tempo; the dynamics, timbre, and tonality do not change; the rhythms are regular, with no accented or syncopated beats; and it tends to employ string or woodwind instruments or vocalization. Above all, for the people who enjoy it, sedate music fosters positive associations, which enhance the relaxation response.

INSTRUCTIONS FOR PROGRESSIVE RELAXATION [1]

Sixteen Muscle Groups

Begin the progressive relaxation by dimming the lights and eliminating all distractions in the room and in yourself (e.g., go to the bathroom, turn off the telephone, put out your pet, close the door). Make sure that your clothing is loose and unrestrictive. If your clothing is restrictive, unbutton the top one or two buttons of your shirt or blouse, unbutton your sleeves, unfasten your belt, or slip off your shoes. Eliminate any other physical discomforts (e.g., make sure that you are sufficiently warm or cool). Begin your music. Position yourself in a chair or on a bed where you can be comfortable. For best results, position yourself on your back; however, it is not essential to do so.

Sit or lie quietly for a few minutes and listen to the music. (At this point, the music should not be accompanied by instruction. Focus your thoughts on the exercises ahead.) The music sets the tone for the progressive relaxation and can cause the effects of the relaxation ex-

---

[1] The three sets of instructions in Appendix A are based on sequences of muscle groups presented by Snyder (1985).

ercise to be more pronounced. Begin the progressive relaxation technique on the dominant side of the body. If you are right-handed, your right side is your dominant side. If you are left-handed, your left side is dominant. Hold tight each muscle group, excluding the muscles of the feet, for 1–7 seconds (Snyder, 1985). When the instructions ask you to tense the muscles, tighten the muscles. When the instructions ask you to relax the muscles, release the muscle tension. Avoid tight tensing of muscles as this could cause injury.

Set 1

Rest your elbows on the arms of the chair or at your sides if you are lying on a bed. Raise your forearm and make a tight fist. Hold it. Relax it. Notice the difference in the way the muscles in your hand and forearm felt between when your tensed them and when you relaxed them. Make another tight fist with the same hand. Hold it. Relax it. Feel the release of tension.

Set 2

With your elbows resting on the arms of the chair or at your sides, push your elbow down into the cushion. Hold it. Relax it. Again, notice the difference in the feeling in your muscles between when you pushed your elbow down–tense–and when you relaxed it. Repeat the elbow push. Hold it. Relax it.

Set 3

Now repeat the fist tightening and the elbow push using your nondominant hand and arm. Rest your elbows on the arms of the chair, or at your sides if you are lying on a bed. Raise your forearm and make a tight fist. Hold it. Relax it. Notice the difference in the way the muscles in your hand and forearm felt between when you tensed them and when you relaxed them. Make another tight fist with the same hand. Hold it. Relax it. Feel the release of tension.

Set 4

With your elbows resting on the arms of the chair or at your sides, push your nondominant elbow down into the cushion. Hold it. Relax it. Notice the difference in the feeling in your muscles between when you pushed your elbow down–tensed–and when you relaxed it.

Repeat the elbow push. Hold it. Relax it. Enjoy the release of tension that you feel.

Set 5

In sets 5–7, you will tense and relax the muscles of your head. Begin by tensing your forehead muscles. To do this, lift your eyebrows as high as possible. Hold it. Relax your forehead. Repeat the eyebrow lift. Lift the eyebrows. Hold the lift, and relax your forehead. Feel the release of the tension in your forehead muscles.

Set 6

To relax the muscles of your cheeks around your nose and your eyes, you will wrinkle your nose and squint your eyes simultaneously. Wrinkle and squint. Hold it. Relax your nose and eye muscles. Repeat the wrinkle and squint. Hold it. Now, relax your face.

Set 7

Next, we will complete the facial muscle relaxation by working the lower face and jaw muscles. This relaxation technique requires you to clench your teeth as you pull back the corners of your mouth. Bite down and pull the corners of your mouth back. Hold it, and now relax. Notice that your facial muscles feel more relaxed after you have held and then released the muscle tension. Repeat by biting down and pulling back the corners of your mouth. Hold it and relax. You should feel relief from facial muscle tension. Pause for a moment and enjoy the release. (Allow a few seconds before proceeding to muscle set 8.)

Set 8

In set 8 you will be working your neck muscles. Pull your chin down to your chest, but do not let it touch your chest. Hold the stretch. Release your neck muscles. Stretch your neck muscles again. Hold the stretch and relax. It is wonderful to relieve the tension in your face and neck muscles. Take a moment to feel the release of tension. (Allow yourself a few seconds before proceeding to muscle set 9.)

Set 9

You will now relieve the tension in your chest, shoulder, and upper back muscles. Take a deep breath and hold it. Push your shoulder blades together. Let go and relax. Repeat the shoulder blade press. Now, release and relax. Notice how your body feels. It may feel heavy because you are much more relaxed than you felt when the relaxation began.

Set 10

In set 10 you will contract, or tighten, the muscles in your abdomen (the "abs"). To tighten these muscles, pull them in as if you are trying to protect them. Contract the abs. Hold the contraction and then relax. Repeat the contraction. Hold it. Relax your abs. Enjoy the tension release. Notice the change between the way your abdomen muscles felt before you tightened them and the way they felt after you released them.

Set 11

Next, you will relax the thigh muscles on your dominant side. (Remember that if you are right-handed, your right leg is your dominant leg. If you are left-handed, your left leg is your dominant leg.) To relax your thigh muscles when seated in a chair, lift your leg and hold it out straight. Do not point your toes. To relax your thigh muscles when lying on a bed, lift your leg until your heel is several inches off the bed. Hold your leg up until you are instructed to relax. Lift your leg. Hold it and relax. Repeat the leg lift. Hold it and relax.

Set 12

Using the same leg, we will now flex and stretch the calf muscles. Rest your foot on the floor or on the bed. Point your toes toward you. Hold it and relax. Repeat the stretch. Hold it and relax. Notice that these calf muscles feel more relaxed than those of your other leg.

Sets 13 and 14

Switching to your nondominant leg, repeat sets 11 and 12.

Set 15

The relaxation exercises are almost over. You should notice a dramatic difference from the way you felt when you first began the exercises. Return your focus to the foot on your dominant side. You will tense the calf muscles by pointing your toes down. To avoid a foot cramp, hold the stretch for less time (5 seconds) than the stretch of the other muscles. If you start to feel uncomfortable, please stop. Point your toes downward. Hold it and relax. Repeat the toe point. Hold it and relax.

Set 16

Using your nondominant leg, repeat set 15. Point the toes. Hold it (no more than 5 seconds) and relax. Repeat the toe point. Hold it and relax.

You have completed the progression through the 16 muscle groups. If you feel that any of your muscles are still tense, stretch and relax the specific muscle groups one more time. Then take some time to enjoy the relaxation you feel. Stay in position and allow yourself to listen to the music. (Omit the following procedure if the relaxation approach is used to invoke sleep.) It will take some time to prepare your body to move after you have relaxed. Avoid becoming dizzy by sitting up and moving slowly. Allow enough time to adjust to your regular level of activity while you appreciate the relief from tension that you feel. Move your arms and legs gently. After a few moments, sit up and hold your sitting position for 2–3 minutes to allow your blood pressure to resume its normal level.

Seven Muscle Groups

The 7 muscle groups progressive relaxation technique is similar to the 16 muscle groups technique, except that this technique combines several muscle groups simultaneously.

Begin the progressive relaxation by dimming the lights and eliminating all distractions in the room and in yourself (e.g., go to the bathroom, turn off the telephone, put out your pet, close the door). Make sure that your clothing is loose and unrestrictive. If your clothing is restrictive, unbutton the top one or two buttons of your shirt or blouse, unbutton your sleeves, unfasten your belt, or slip off your shoes. Eliminate any other physical discomforts (e.g., make sure that you are sufficiently warm or cool). Begin your music. Position yourself in a chair or on a bed where you can be comfortable. For best results, position yourself on your back; however, it is not essential to do so.

Sit or lie quietly for a few minutes and listen to the music. (At this point, the music should not be accompanied by instruction. Focus your thoughts on the exercises ahead.) The music sets the tone for the progressive relaxation and can cause the effects of the relaxation exercise to be more pronounced. Hold tight each muscle group, excluding the muscle of the feet, for 1–7 seconds (Snyder, 1985). When the instructions ask you to tense the muscles, tighten the muscles. When the instructions ask you to relax the muscles, release the muscle tension. Avoid tight tensing of muscles as this could cause injury.

Set 1

Begin the progressive relaxation with your dominant hand, forearm, and bicep. If you are right-handed, your right hand and arm are dominant. If you are left-handed, your left hand and arm are dominant. Rest your elbows on the arms of the chair, or at your sides if you are lying on a bed. Now, clench your fist as you push your elbow into the arm of the chair or into the mattress. Hold it and relax. Repeat this movement. Hold it and relax. Notice the reduction in muscle tension in your hand and arm.

Set 2

Using your nondominant hand and arm, repeat set 1. Enjoy the release of tension in both sets of hands and arms.

Set 3

Next, relax the muscles of your face. Wrinkle your nose, squint your eyes, clench your teeth, and pull back the corners of your mouth all at once. Hold it and relax. Repeat the facial relaxation. Hold it and relax. Pause for a moment and feel the release of tension in your face.

Set 4

In set 4, relax your neck muscles. Pull your chin down to your chest, but do not let it touch your chest. Hold it and relax. Repeat the neck muscle stretch. Hold it and relax.

Set 5

Set 5 combines the muscles of your back and your abdomen. Take a slow, deep breath, push back your shoulder blades, and pull in your abdominal muscles. Hold this position and now relax. Repeat these movements. Hold the tension and relax. Take a moment to enjoy the release of tension.

Set 6

Now, if you are seated, lift your dominant leg until it is held straight out from your body. If you are lying on a bed, lift your leg until your heel is a few inches off the mattress. As you lift, point your toes toward you. Hold it and relax. Try it once again. Hold it and relax.

Set 7

For the final set, switch to your nondominant leg. Lift your leg and point your toes toward you. Hold it and relax. Repeat the leg lift and toe point. Hold it and relax.

You have completed the progression through the seven muscle groups. If you feel that any of your muscles are still tense, stretch and relax the specific muscle groups one more time. Then take some time to enjoy the relaxation you feel. Stay in position and allow yourself to listen to the music. (Omit the following procedure if the relaxation approach is used to invoke sleep.) It will take some time to prepare your body to move after you have relaxed. Avoid becoming dizzy by sitting up and moving slowly. Allow enough time to adjust to your regular level of activity while you appreciate the relief from tension that you feel. Move your arms and legs gently. After a few moments, sit up and hold your sitting position for 2–3 minutes to allow your blood pressure to resume its normal level.

Four Muscle Groups

The 4 muscle groups progressive relaxation technique is similar to the 16 muscle groups technique except that this technique combines several muscle groups simultaneously.

Begin the progressive relaxation by dimming the lights and eliminating all distractions in the room and in yourself (e.g., go to the bathroom, turn off the telephone, put out your pet, close the door). Make sure that your clothing is loose and unrestrictive. If your clothing is restrictive, unbutton the top one or two buttons of your shirt or blouse, unbutton your sleeves, unfasten your belt, or slip off your shoes. Eliminate any other physical discomforts (e.g., make sure that you are sufficiently warm or cool). Begin your music. Position yourself in a chair or on a bed where you can be comfortable. For best results, position yourself on your back; however, it is not essential to do so.

Sit or lie quietly for a few minutes and listen to the music. (At this point the music should not be accompanied by instruction. Focus your thoughts on the exercises ahead.) The music sets the tone for the progressive relaxation and can cause the effects of the relaxation exercise to be more pronounced. Hold tight each muscle group, excluding the muscles of the feet, for 1–7 seconds (Snyder, 1985). When the instructions ask you to tense the muscles, tighten the muscles. When the instructions ask you to relax the muscles, release the muscle tension. Avoid tight tensing of muscles as this could cause injury.

Set 1

Begin the progressive relaxation with both hands, forearms, and biceps at once. Rest your elbows on the arms of the chair, or at your sides if you are lying on a bed. Now, clench both of your fists as you push your elbows down into the arms of the chair or into the mattress. Hold it and relax. Repeat the movement. Hold it and relax. Notice the reduction in muscle tension in your hands and arms.

Set 2

In set 2, simultaneously wrinkle your nose, squint your eyes, clench your teeth, pull back the corners of your mouth, and pull your chin down to your chest without touching it. Hold it and relax. Now, repeat the head and neck movements. Hold it and relax. Pause for a moment to feel and enjoy the release of tension.

Set 3

Set 3 combines the muscles of your back and your abdomen. Take a slow, deep breath, push back your shoulder blades, and pull in your abdominal muscles. Hold this position and now relax. Repeat the tensing, hold it, and relax. Notice how good it feels.

Set 4

If you are seated, lift both legs until they are held straight out from your body. If you are lying on a bed, lift your legs until your heels are a few inches off the bed. (Note: You may find it very difficult to raise both legs at one time. This exercise can be modified to begin with the dominant leg and move to the nondominant leg, as in the instructions for the seven muscle groups technique.) As you lift, point your toes toward you. Hold it and relax. Now, repeat the movement. Hold it and relax. Be sure to feel the release of tension.

You have completed the progression through the muscle groups. If you feel that any of your muscles are still tense, stretch and relax the specific muscle groups one more time. Then take some time to enjoy the relaxation you feel. Stay in position and allow yourself to listen to the music. (Omit the following procedure if the relaxation approach is used to invoke sleep.) It will take some time to prepare your body to move after you have relaxed. Avoid becoming dizzy by sitting up and moving slowly. Allow enough time to adjust to your regular level of activity while you appreciate the relief from tension that you feel. Move your arms and legs gently. After a few moments, sit up and hold your sitting position for 2–3 minutes to allow your blood pressure to resume its normal level.

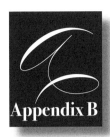

Appendix B

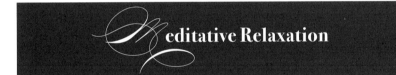

Meditative Relaxation

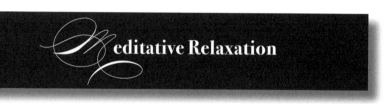

A great deal of music is marketed for relaxation purposes. Music for relaxation and stress management is commonly found in any music retail store. Some of this music may be very good for you, but some may be disquieting and uncomfortable. The author suggests trying different musical selections of all styles to determine which music is most suitable.

In selecting music, be aware of the ways in which you or your care recipient responds to the music. The music should engender quietude and should not stimulate any physical movement or agitation whatsoever (e.g., toe tapping, hand clapping, swaying, and dancing). Music that is melodic, with unaccented and unsyncopated rhythms, using strings, woodwinds, or synthesizer rather than brass and percussion should be selected. However, exceptions can be made.

The music must be compatible with your rhythm of breathing or that of your care recipient. The tempo of the music should be neither faster nor slower than your usual rate of inhalation and exhalation. To determine rhythmic compatibility between a music selections and your breathing pattern, breathe slowly and deeply while you listen. If you feel that the music increases your rate of breathing or if it tends to force you to breathe uncomfortably slowly, then it is the wrong music for you to use. Try another selection.

Not only should the music and your breathing be rhythmically compatible, but the music should also bring memories of and associations with comfort or general feelings of well-being. If you do not feel comfort and calm when you listen to a particular selection, make another choice.

The best way to find the music that suits you is to listen to several pieces, breathe along with them, and judge for yourself. Remember that the music that someone else recommends may or may not be music that works well for you.

The instructions for meditative relaxation can be read by someone who is able to stay with an individual throughout the meditation session. The instructions can also be recorded for use at any time. After some practice with the instructions, you can adapt them to meet individual preferences and time allowances. Some individuals may wish to abandon the instructions and try self-initiated relaxation exercises. The instructions for conducting meditative relaxation follow.

Begin the meditative relaxation with your meditative music.

Your music should promote calm and quiet in you. When you hear it, you should feel comfort and peace. As your music plays, it is important to prepare your environment to facilitate meditation. Dim the lights and eliminate all distractions in the room and in yourself (e.g., go to the bathroom, turn off the telephone, put out your pet, close the door). Make sure that your clothing is loose and unrestrictive. If your clothing is restrictive, unbutton the top one or two buttons of your shirt or blouse, unbutton your sleeves, unfasten your belt, or slip off your shoes. Eliminate any other physical discomforts (e.g., make sure that you are sufficiently warm or cool). Position yourself in a chair or on a bed where you can be comfortable. For best results, position yourself on your back; however, it is not essential to do so.

Once you are in a comfortable position, close your eyes. Listen to your music and inhale and exhale in time with it. As you exhale, let go of the tension. Allow the music to draw out the tension from your body as you continue to exhale any tightness. (Allow several moments for breathing. The duration depends on the ability to remain focused on the activity. If rhythmic breathing is interrupted or discontinued or if there is some other indication of inattentiveness, the instructions should include more patter that directs attention to the breathing while the subject concentrates on releasing tension.) Continue to breathe deeply and slowly. Allow your abdomen to expand (rise) as you inhale and to contract (fall) as you exhale. Let your breathing be natural as you exhale your tension. (Allow a minimum of 20 seconds for breathing.) As you exhale, you may also want to repeat a word or a short (one or two words) phrase silently to yourself. This "mantra" can be any word or phrase that brings you comfort, peace, or calm. It can be a word or phrase associated with your spiritual beliefs.

Meditative relaxation works for any part of the body that feels tense. You can start with your face, and move slowly down your body to your shoulders, back, lower back, buttocks, thighs, calves, and feet. You may also focus only on the area where you feel the greatest amount of tension and meditate on the tension drawing away from your body. (Allow a few moments to work with this concept—a minimum of 20 seconds to a maximum of several minutes depending on involvement and attention focus. This approach can take a while in people who find it appealing.)

Continue to breathe deeply and slowly with the music. You may begin to identify your feeling of relaxation. For some people, it is a feeling of heaviness and warmth. For others, it is a feeling of numbness and coolness. If you do not feel any sensation in any part of you, try to focus your attention on that area.

Exhale the tension and feel it being drawn away from your body. It will take some time to prepare your body to move after you have relaxed. Avoid becoming dizzy by sitting up and moving slowly. Allow enough time to adjust to your regular level of activity while you appreciate the relief from tension that you feel. Move your arms and legs gently. After a few moments, sit up and hold your sitting position for 2–3 minutes to allow your blood pressure to resume its normal level.

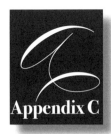

Appendix C

Visualization in Relaxation

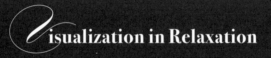

Visualization in Relaxation

When developing one's own imagery for visualization in relaxation, the source material used may be anything that is positive and enjoyable. This could include, for example, picturing oneself in a favorite place doing a favorite activity, either alone or with loved ones. You may also choose to picture scenes related to spiritual beliefs, such as seeing oneself in an encounter with God or his or her higher power. Such an encounter may be characterized by a personal, protective relationship with a strong humanlike figure who has certain features (e.g., arms that wrap gently around the person to caress and hold him or her, physical characteristics such as kindly eyes or a large physical presence that represent comfort and safety, clothes that are soft to the touch) that foster feelings of peace and consolation. For some people, this figure may be a father figure, yet for others the figure may be a mother figure. Visualizations may include being held, leaning one's head upon the figure's chest, and hearing the figure's soft, quiet heartbeat.

If this image does not appeal, one should try to find an image that promotes a particular sensory stimulus that aids in the release of physical tension and relaxation. This image may be a warm, soft light that draws the tension from various parts of the body as the person thinks about moving it from place to place on the body. Some people may not find a warm light comforting and may find relief from visualizing a cool, blue light. Other people may visualize an image that changes as they become relaxed (e.g., a bright orange ball may become smaller and duller until it turns to a pinpoint of beige and then disappears completely as the tension dissipates).

Whatever visualization approach is used, it is important for it to be personally effective as determined by the individual. Be sure that any suggested images or visualizations are compatible with the person's or one's own experiences of comfort. If an image is not comfortable and appealing, it will not enhance the relaxation response. In addition, it is important to use only one type of imagery at a time. If there is too much stimulation, none of it will be helpful. Be careful when making your image selection.

Music can be used to enhance visualization. The music can be associated with a particular picture or can tend to evoke pleasant thoughts that can be developed into visualization imagery. This music must promote comfort and quiet, not movement (e.g., toe tapping).

Music can be the sole stimulus in the environment as one visualizes. However, if concentration is difficult because the only stimulus is music, an audio recording of the instructions can be made to be played while listening to the music once the most effective approach is determined. (Adding the voice-over requires a player for the music, a microphone, and a recording device that can record both the music and the spoken cues that lead one through the visualization.) The instructions for conducting visualization follow.

Begin the visualization by dimming the lights and eliminating all distractions in the room and in yourself (e.g., go to the bathroom, turn off the telephone, put out your pet, close the door). Make sure that your clothing is loose and unrestrictive. If your clothing is restrictive, unbutton the top one or two buttons of your shirt or blouse, unbutton your sleeves, unfasten your belt, or slip off your shoes. Eliminate any other physical discomforts (e.g., make sure that you are sufficiently warm or cool). Position yourself in a chair or on a bed where you can be comfortable. For best results, position yourself on your back; however, it is not essential to do so.

Once you are comfortable, begin your music. Remember that this music must be calming and peaceful. You may find a particular type of music helpful in visualization under certain circumstances, but at other times, the same music may not seem effective at all. Pay particular attention to whether your responses to the music are desirable.

As you listen to your music, begin to inhale and exhale deeply. It may be possible to match your breathing to the tempo of your calming music. Be careful not to hyperventilate. You may wish to close your eyes as you begin to visualize the image you have selected. As you visualize the image, let go of your tension. Visualize the image for as long as you like. If you find it difficult to use the imagery to relax your entire body, use an image that allows you to focus on only one area at a time. Begin the visualization with the area of your body that feels the most tension. Focus the image on that area while listening to the music and breathing in and out until the tension begins to subside. It may not be possible to remove all of your tension completely, but you will likely sense a release of tension as you move the image around your body.

It will take some time to prepare your body to move after you have relaxed. Avoid becoming dizzy by sitting up and moving slowly. Allow enough time to adjust to your regular level of activity while you appreciate the relief from tension that you feel. Move your arms and legs gently. After a few moments, sit up and hold your sitting position for 2–3 minutes to allow your blood pressure to resume its normal level.

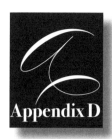

Appendix D

Jaw Drop Relaxation Technique

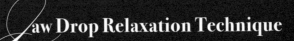

The jaw drop technique is very simple and requires little practice. It is effective with people who have moderate to severe pain and can be implemented quickly, especially if it is rehearsed prior to feeling any sensations of pain (McCaffery & Pasero, 1999). The effects of the jaw drop technique may be enhanced with music that is selected to suit individual tastes and comfort levels. Therefore, it is important for each person to select music that promotes comfort. Familiar music is a good choice, unless so many memories are associated with it that it distracts the individual from the relaxation. Familiar or unfamiliar, the music must promote feelings of calm and quiet and must not encourage movement (e.g., toe tapping). Because it involves relaxing the tongue, the technique must be used only when the head is somewhat elevated in order to avoid blocking the airways. The instructions for conducting the jaw drop relaxation technique follow.

Begin the relaxation by dimming the lights and eliminating all distractions in the room and in yourself (e.g., go to the bathroom, turn off the telephone, put out your pet, close the door). Make sure that your clothing is loose and unrestrictive. If your clothing is restrictive, unbutton the top one or two buttons of your shirt or blouse, unbutton your sleeves, unfasten your belt, or slip off your shoes. Eliminate any other physical discomforts (e.g., make sure that you are sufficiently warm or cool). Position yourself in a chair or on a bed where you can be comfortable. For best results, position yourself on your back; however, it is not essential to do so.

Start your music and very slowly inhale and exhale in time to the rhythm. Drop your jaw slightly, as if you are about to yawn. Allow your tongue to drop into the bottom of your mouth. To do this, place the tip of your tongue at the base of your bottom teeth and let go of the back of your tongue. Let your tongue spread over the bottom of your mouth cavity. Let your lips become soft and release any tension in the corners of your mouth. Slowly inhale and exhale, allowing your lungs to fill and empty at your own pace. Clear your mind of all thoughts. Do not attempt to speak. Continue to focus on relaxing your jaw, tongue, and lips as you slowly and rhythmically inhale and exhale. Once you feel relaxed, listen to your music for as long as you like.

It will take some time to prepare your body to move after you have relaxed. Avoid becoming dizzy by sitting up and moving slowly. Allow enough time to adjust to your regular level of activity while you appreciate the relief from tension that you feel. Move your arms and legs gently. After a few moments, sit up and hold your sitting position for 2–3 minutes to allow your blood pressure to resume its normal level.

REFERENCES

Heide, F. J., & Borkovec, T. D. (1984). Relaxation-induced anxiety: Mechanisms and theoretical implications. *Behavior Research in Therapy*, 22(1), 1–12.

McCaffery, M., & Pasero, C. (1999). *Pain: Clinical manual* (2nd ed.). St. Louis, MO: Mosby.

Pender, N. J., Murdaugh, C., & Parsons, M. A. (2006). *Health promotion in nursing practice* (5th ed.). Upper Saddle River, NJ: Prentice-Hall Health.

Snyder, M. (1985). *Independent nursing interventions*. New York: John Wiley & Sons.

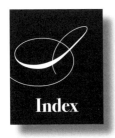

Index